Global Medical Physics

Global Medical Physics: A Guide for International Collaboration provides essential guidance for medical physicists and other healthcare professionals seeking to collaborate internationally in clinical, educational, and research settings.

With the growing interest in global health initiatives, this book addresses the complexities of working across diverse healthcare environments, particularly in low-resource settings. It explores the increasing role of medical physicists in international education, training, and research collaborations, emphasizing the importance of cultural competence, ethical considerations, and overcoming technological barriers.

Features:

- Explores the expanding role of medical physicists in global health education, training, and research

- Examines challenges in cross-cultural collaboration, including ethical concerns, technological limitations, and language barriers

- Discusses the rise of "big data" and artificial intelligence applications in international medical physics

- Provides practical strategies for successful global health partnerships, including guidelines for Short-Term Experiences in Global Health (STEGHs)

- Includes contributions from 34 experts across 21 countries, representing diverse perspectives from both high- and low-resource settings

- Features clear chapter objectives and summaries, with key recommendations compiled into a separate reference guide

- Developed as an open-source resource to ensure accessibility for professionals in lower-income regions

This book is an essential resource for medical physicists at all career stages, including graduate students, residents, educators, and experienced professionals. It is also valuable for healthcare providers, researchers, and policymakers interested in global health initiatives, fostering effective international collaborations in medical physics.

Global Medical Physics

A Guide for International Collaboration

Edited by
Jacob Van Dyk

CRC Press
Taylor & Francis Group
Boca Raton London New York

CRC Press is an imprint of the
Taylor & Francis Group, an **informa** business

Designed cover image: Shutterstock

First edition published 2026
by CRC Press
2385 NW Executive Center Drive, Suite 320, Boca Raton FL 33431

and by CRC Press
4 Park Square, Milton Park, Abingdon, Oxon, OX14 4RN

CRC Press is an imprint of Taylor & Francis Group, LLC

ISBN: 978-1-032-86487-7 (hbk)
ISBN: 978-1-032-86489-1 (pbk)
ISBN: 978-1-003-52774-9 (ebk)

DOI: 10.1201/9781003527749

Typeset in Minion
by Deanta Global Publishing Services, Chennai, India

Access the Support Material: www.routledge.com/9781032864877

*To all those Medical Physicists who contribute their
knowledge, experience, time, and energy in support of global
medical physics activities. It is through joint collaborations
and partnerships that "together we can do so much."*

Contents

Preface

THERE IS A GROWING interest among medical physicists and other medical professionals to provide education, training, and consulting support to their counterparts in less-resourced environments. Furthermore, there is an increased enthusiasm for fostering international research collaborations, partly in response to the generation of "big data" and the corresponding applications using artificial intelligence (AI). This interest is further supported by the number of related publications in the peer-reviewed literature. A PubMed search up to the end of 2024 on "Global Health in Medical Physics" showed a clear increase from 13/year in 2012 to 387/year in 2024. There continues to be a similar growth in other areas of Global Health as well. Moreover, the American Association of Physicists in Medicine (AAPM) has updated its organizational structure within the last few years with a new *International Council* specifically to collaborate and provide support in the international medical physics world. Similarly, in 2018, the American Physical Society (APS) developed a report on expanding international engagement. A comparable increase in emphasis on international activities is taking place in various radiation therapy and diagnostic imaging related societies around the globe. In a global health interest survey performed by the Association of Residents in Radiation Oncology (ARRO) and published in 2014, 90% of the responders indicated an interest in a global health residency educational experience in radiation oncology and 80% indicated a wish to incorporate international work in their future career. This was followed a year later by an opinion piece making the case for elective international rotations during their residency training for both radiation oncologists and medical physicists.

These types of international engagements have become increasingly prevalent especially over the last decade, and many of these activities are now known as Short-Term Experiences in Global Health (STEGHs). However, being professionally trained and working in one societal context does not necessarily provide the skills needed to participate in other cultural contexts or lower-resource environments. Indeed, in some instances, these STEGHs can be counterproductive and even harmful. Books have been written on "when helping hurts." In addition, international collaborations in the research world also have their unique considerations. With international involvement, successful engagement may be obstructed by multiple barriers, ranging from cultural, to language, to ethical, to internet and technology limitations.

The *main purpose of this book* is to provide guidance, primarily to medical physicists, in both low- and high-income countries on issues related to partnering with colleagues in different country settings, especially in the clinical and educational medical physics circles, and also in research and academic environments. This book may be of value to other professional and scientific groups as well, since many of the topics are generic and not only applicable to medical physicists. The book is geared at multiple levels of interest and expertise ranging from graduate students, to residents in training, to fully experienced medical physicists. Potential barriers and concerns as well as guidelines for success are addressed.

Each chapter includes clear objectives at the beginning and a summary with recommendations at the end. These objectives, summaries, and recommendations are collated as a separate document useful as an abbreviated guide for those involved in global medical physics activities.

The book is developed as an open-source guide to make it readily available to everyone, including those living in lower-income societies.

The contributing authors were selected for their expertise and experience in global health and medical physics activities. Furthermore, all the primary authors were invited to find collaborators from another part of the globe, thus exemplifying true international collaborations and enhancing the global medical physics contents. The 34 authors and co-authors represent experiences from 21 countries, with 11 being from low- to middle-income countries.

My hope is that the chapters provided by the contributors to this book will enhance the global health experiences for all those who are involved in international partnerships. To quote Helen Keller, "Alone we can do so little; together we can do so much." This working together is greatly enhanced by being educated to understand our partners' circumstances, environment, and culture. All these contribute to working together so we can do so much.

Acknowledgements

This book has been made possible through the enthusiastic support of the following:

All the authors and co-authors who have taken the time out of their busyness to contribute chapters in support of their global medical physics collaborations.

The financial contributors who have made this book available as an open-access text so that it could be equally available to all medical physicists around the globe.

CRC Press/Taylor & Francis for enthusiastically accepting this book proposal.

The multiple staff members associated with CRC Press/Taylor & Francis for providing their support and bringing this book to completion.

Christine Van Dyk, my dear wife, who continues to provide unmitigated support for my enthusiastic projects which take significant time even in our retirement years.

About the Editor

JACOB (JAKE) VAN DYK is Professor Emeritus of Oncology and Medical Biophysics at Western University, London, Ontario, Canada, and former Manager of Physics and Engineering at the London Regional Cancer Program (LRCP). He has more than 40 years of experience in the practical facets of radiation oncology physics, with 24 years at the Princess Margaret Hospital (PMH) in Toronto and 15 years at the LRCP. With a leave-of-absence in 1974–1975, he worked as the acting head of physics at the Centre de Radiothérapy, Hôpital Cantonal de Génève, in Geneva, Switzerland. From 2009 to 2011, he was employed as a professional expert and consultant at the International Atomic Energy Agency (IAEA) in Vienna, Austria. His research has yielded over 200 publications along with four unique volumes of *The Modern Technology of Radiation Oncology: A Compendium for Medical Physicists and Radiation Oncologists*. He also published *True Tales of Medical Physics: Insights into a Life-Saving Specialty*, a book giving a wide range of perspectives on medical physics to a broader, non-scientific audience. He has lectured in over 41 countries. He was the main founder of *Medical Physics for World Benefit* (www.mpwb .org), an organization devoted to supporting medical physics activities, largely by training and mentoring, especially for lower-income settings. He is the recipient of multiple awards including:

- The William D. Coolidge Gold Medal (2022), the highest award given by the American Association of Physicists in Medicine (AAPM) "recognizing an eminent career in Medical Physics."

- The International Day of Medical Physics (IDMP) Award (2019) for "promoting medical physics to a larger audience and highlighting the contributions medical physicists make for patient care." Awarded by the International Organization for Medical Physics.

- Honorary Doctor of Science (honoris causa) degree granted at Western University's MD Convocation, London, Ontario, Canada (2014) "for advancing the field of medical physics, specifically, the safe use of therapeutic radiation for the treatment of cancer. In so doing, he has touched the lives of millions of people in Canada and around the world."

- Selected by the International Organization for Medical Physics (IOMP) as one out of 50 medical physicists "who have made an outstanding contribution to the advancement of medical physics over the last 50 years." This recognition was given as part of IOMP's 50th anniversary in 2013.

- Awarded the inaugural *Fellow of the Canadian Organization of Medical Physicists (FCOMP)* in 2013 in recognition of "his significant contribution to the organization and to the field of Medical Physics in Canada."

- *Canadian Organization of Medical Physicists (COMP) Gold Medal* (2013). This is the highest honour that COMP bestows on one of its members in recognition of an outstanding career as a medical physicist who has worked mainly in Canada.

- Elected *Fellow of the American Association of Physicists in Medicine* in recognition of distinguished contributions to the field of Medical Physics (1997).

Contributors

May Abdel-Wahab
Division of Human Health,
  Department of Nuclear Sciences
  and Applications
International Atomic Energy
  Agency
Vienna, Austria

Akshaya Neil Arya
Department of Environment and
  Resource Studies now School of
  Public Health Sciences
University of Waterloo
Waterloo, ON, Canada

Stephen M. Avery
Department of Environment and
  Resource Studies now School of
  Public Health Sciences
University of Waterloo
Waterloo, ON, Canada

Godfrey Azangwe
Dosimetry and Medical Radiation
  Physics, Division of Human
  Health
International Atomic Energy
  Agency (IAEA)
Vienna, Austria

Eva Bezak
Allied Health & Human
  Performance
University of South Australia
Adelaide, Australia
and
Department of Physics
University of Adelaide
Adelaide, Australia

Mauro Carrara
Dosimetry and Medical Radiation
  Physics, Division of Human
  Health
International Atomic Energy
  Agency (IAEA)
Vienna, Austria

Arun Chougule
Swasthya Kalyan Group of
  Institutions
Jaipur, Rajasthan, India

Laurence Court
Department of Radiation
  Physics
University of Texas MD Anderson
  Cancer Center
Houston, TX, USA

Andre Dekker
Maastro Clinic
Maastricht University Medical
    Centre
Maastricht, The Netherlands

Jennifer Dent
BIO Ventures for Global Health
Seattle, WA, USA

Manjit Dosanjh
Department of Physics
University of Oxford
Oxford, United Kingdom
and
Accelerator Technology Sector
CERN
Geneva, Switzerland

Denis Dudas
Faculty of Nuclear Sciences and
    Physical Engineering
Czech Technical University in Prague
Prague, Czechia

Martin Ebert
Sir Charles Gairdner Hospital
Nedlands, Western Australia,
    Australia
and
University of Western Australia
Perth, Western Australia, Australia

K. Ruwani M. Fernando
Department of Machine Learning
H. Lee Moffitt Cancer Center &
    Research Institute
Tampa, FL

Katy Graef
Programs at BIO Ventures for
    Global Health
Seattle, WA, USA

Francis Hasford
Radiological and Medical
    Sciences Research Institute
Ghana Atomic Energy
    Commission
Accra, Ghana

Robert Jeraj
University of Wisconsin
Madison, WI, USA
and
University of Ljubljana
Slovenia

Mary Joan
Christian Medical College and
    Hospital
Ludhiana, Punjab, India

Cathyryne Manner
BIO Ventures for Global Health
Seattle, WA, USA

Loredana Marcu
Allied Health & Human
    Performance
University of South Australia
Adelaide, Australia
and
Faculty of Informatics & Science
University of Oradea
Oradea, Romania

Lisbeth Cordero Mendez
Applied Radiation Biology and
    Radiotherapy
Division of Human Health
International Atomic Energy
    Agency (IAEA)
Vienna, Austria

Mauro Namias
Fundación Centro Diagnóstico
    Nuclear
Buenos Aires, Argentina

Issam El Naqa
Department of Machine Learning
H. Lee Moffitt Cancer Center &
    Research Institute
Tampa, FL, USA

Kwan Hoong Ng
Department of Biomedical
    Imaging, Faculty of Medicine
Universiti Malaya
Kuala Lumpur, Malaysia

Dipesh Niraula
Department of Machine Learning
H. Lee Moffitt Cancer Center &
    Research Institute,
Tampa, FL, USA

Loreh Peter Onyango
Kenyatta University Teaching,
    Referral & Research Hospital
Nairobi, Kenya

Stephanie A. Parker
Radiation Oncology
Wake Forest Baptist Health High
    Point Medical Center
High Point, NC, USA

Alfredo Polo
Technical Cooperation and
    Capacity Development
City Cancer Challenge
Geneva, Switzerland

Dario Sanz
Instituto Balseiro
San Carlos de Bariloche, Rio
    Negro. Argentina

William Shaw
Department of Medical
    Physics
University of the Free State
Bloemfontein, South Africa

Ana Maria Marques da Silva
Hospital das Clínicas, Faculdade
    de Medicina
Universidade de São Paulo
São Paulo, Brazil

Steinar Stapnes
Accelerator Technology Sector
CERN
Geneva, Switzerland

Egor Titovich
Dosimetry and Medical Radiation
    Physics, Division of Human
    Health
International Atomic Energy
    Agency (IAEA)
Vienna, Austria

Iyobosa B. Uwadiae
University College Hospital
Ibadan, Nigeria

Gerald A. White
Medical Physics Services
Colorado Springs, CO, USA

Laurence Wroe
Accelerator Technology Sector
CERN
Geneva, Switzerland

Afua A. Yorke
Radiation Oncology
University of Washington Medical
   Center
Seattle, WA, USA

CHAPTER 1

Introduction to Global Medical Physics

Jacob Van Dyk and Francis Hasford

1.1 CHAPTER OBJECTIVES

- To define specific terms associated with global medical physics activities
- To provide a broad overview of global medical physics
- To describe global medical physics issues and concerns
- To provide a high-level description of international collaboration and outreach considerations
- To provide recommendations on global medical physics activities

1.2 TERMINOLOGY

1.2.1 Medical Physics/Medical Physicist

Medical physics aims to prevent, diagnose, and treat human diseases using physics applications. Medical physicists work in areas like medical imaging, radiotherapy, especially for cancer treatment, cardiology, radiation safety, non-ionizing radiation medical physics, and physics related to physiological measurement. It is also closely aligned with neighbouring sciences such as (Medical or Laser) Biophysics, Biological Physics, and Radiobiology. Medical physicists working in a healthcare setting need appropriate certification to establish their competence to practice independently in one of the subdisciplines.

DOI: 10.1201/9781003527749-1

1

1.2.2 Global Medical Physics

One definition of Global Health is *collaborative trans-national research and action for promoting health for all* [1]. An analogous definition of Global Medical Physics could be *collaborative trans-national research and action for promoting medical physics to benefit health for all.*

1.2.3 International

International refers to activities that involve two or more countries. This can include healthcare along with medical physics–related activities.

1.2.4 Collaboration

The short definition of collaboration is the act or process of voluntarily working together to achieve a common goal. In the global context, collaboration involves efforts among individuals, institutions, or organizations from different geographical locations to share knowledge, resources, and insights for collective learning and progress [2].

1.2.5 Global North, Global South Collaborations

Global North and *Global South* are terms that denote a method of grouping countries based on their defining characteristics regarding socioeconomics and politics. According to the United Nations Conference on Trade and Development (UNCTAD), the developing economies (often referred to as the Global South) broadly comprise Africa, Latin America and the Caribbean, Asia without Israel, Japan, and the Republic of Korea, and Oceania without Australia and New Zealand. Most of the Global South's countries are commonly identified as lacking in their standard of living, which includes having lower incomes, high levels of poverty, high population growth rates, inadequate housing, limited educational opportunities, and deficient health systems, among other issues. Additionally, cities in these countries are characterized by their poor infrastructure. Opposite to the Global South is the Global North, which the UNCTAD describes as broadly comprising Northern America and Europe, Israel, Japan, South Korea, Australia, and New Zealand [3, 4].

A world map of the Global North and the Global South is shown in Figure 1.1.

1.2.6 Colonialism

While there is no clear definition of colonialism, it is often described as "'control by one power over a dependent area or people.' It occurs when one nation subjugates another, conquering its population and exploiting

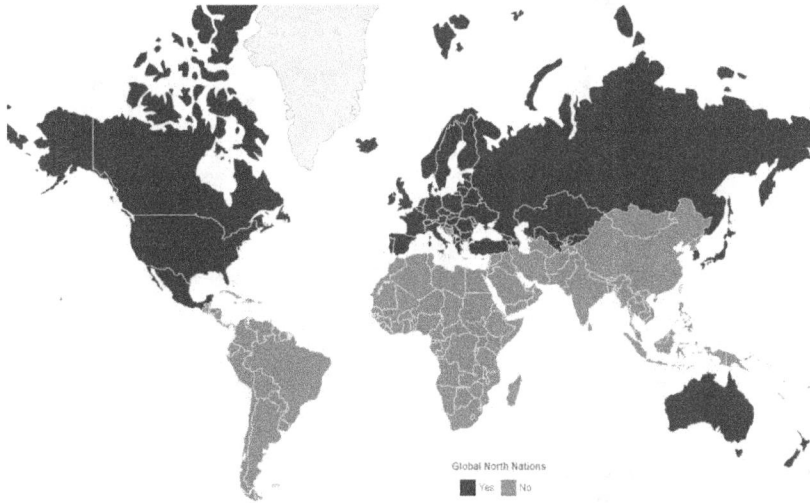

FIGURE 1.1   World map of the Global North and the Global South. Adapted with permission from [5].

it, often while forcing its own language and cultural values upon its people" [6].

1.2.7 Neocolonialism

"The economic and political policies by which a great power indirectly maintains or extends its influence over other areas or people" [7].

1.2.8 Global Health

"An area for study, research, and practice that places a priority on improving health and achieving health equity for all people worldwide [8]."

1.3 GLOBAL MEDICAL PHYSICS WORKFORCE

Medical physics is a global enterprise as summarized by the International Organization for Medical Physics (IOMP) workforce review [9], which indicated that in 2022 there were nearly 30,000 medical physicists in 93 countries, of whom 30% are women and 70% specialize in radiation oncology medical physics. The distribution of medical physicists around the globe is shown in Figure 1.2a, although as shown in Figure 1.2b there is a huge variation in the number of medical physicists per capita, with lower-income countries having the least. Of course, these data are dependent on reporting accuracy. For example, the previously published work from the Federation of African Medical Physics Organizations (FAMPO) put

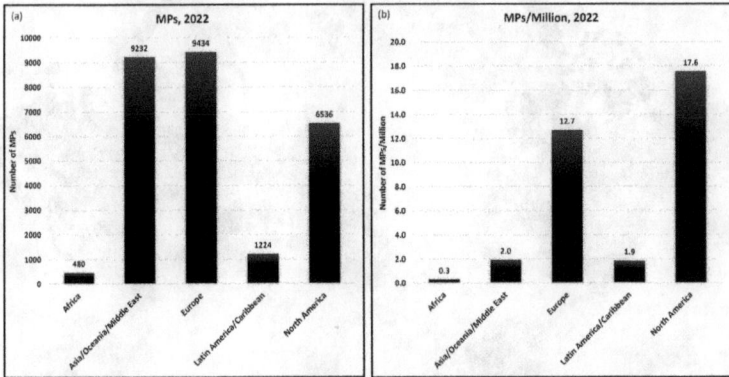

FIGURE 1.2 Distribution of medical physicists (MPs) in major regions of the globe in 2022. (a) Total number of MPs per region, and (b) number of MPs per million population. (Based on data from [9]. We acknowledge Eva Bezak for forwarding the raw data to generate this figure.)

the number of medical physicists in Africa at 1041 [10]. The projection for 2035 is that an additional 30,000 medical physicists will be required [9]. In 2050, about 47,000 medical physicists will be needed in radiation oncology alone [11]. The survey results showed significant variations in the scope and contents of the education and training programmes, with 53% of respondents indicating graduate courses at the master's level [9].

1.4 GLOBAL MEDICAL PHYSICS ISSUES

1.4.1 Workforce Disparities

The disparity in the number of medical physicists per country, as shown in Figure 1.2, is a result of multiple complex factors. It begins with the structure of the healthcare system in a country which is influenced by the wealth of the nation (or the lack thereof). A couple of reports commissioned by Lancet Oncology have shown the dramatic projected needs for medical physicists. The 2015 Commission on expanding radiotherapy [12] projected that an additional 22,000 medical physicists would be required by 2035 if adequate radiotherapy were going to be available at that time. However, for this need to be met, an additional 13,000 MV radiation therapy machines would be required along with 6,500 CT scanners, 30,000 radiation oncologists, and 78,000 radiation therapists (RTTs). While providing fully adequate radiotherapy globally as an idealistic goal, the reality is that the need for a significant increase is clear and that we should position ourselves to address substantial increases. Similarly, the Lancet

Commission [13] on imaging and nuclear medicine identified substantial shortages in equipment and workforce, particularly in low- and middle-income countries (LMICs). The shortage of medical physicists even in today's circumstances was also clearly identified in the 2023 medical physics workforce study [9].

1.4.2 Training Disparities

The requirements for education and training in medical physics are significant, especially for medical physicists aiming to work in clinical environments. While there are variations around the world with respect to both academic and clinical training requirements, generally, there is an expectation of a graduate degree in medical physics or a related discipline at either the master's or PhD level. In addition, for those working in clinical environments, there is an expectation of a period of on-the-job, hands-on training, generally known as a residency programme (or internship or registrar programme in some countries). The most common residency programme consists of two years of clinical training. However, a survey involving 77 countries indicated large variations in times for full university and residency training ranging from three to nine years, with the peak of the distribution being at five years [14]. A more recent survey published in 2023 [15] indicated that a number of multi-national organizations are advocating for harmonization of medical physics education and training across the globe, but that much more work remains to be done.

1.4.3 Disparities in Accreditation and Certification

The requirements for accreditation of academic institutions and clinical departments need to be developed at the national level and would include consideration of human resources, physical resources, equipment, core syllabus suitable for education and training, and quality indicators. As part of the global harmonization process, the International Atomic Energy Agency (IAEA) describes accreditation and certification procedures [16].

Certification could involve written, practical, and oral examinations but could also include other elements depending on the national requirements including satisfactory completion of competencies, maintenance and presentation of a portfolio of best work, and evidence of a scientific publication or conference presentation. Certification is awarded by an authorized body such as a Certification Board, which would likely be made up of senior Clinically Qualified Medical Physicists (CQMPs).

Certification demonstrates the ability of the resident to be an independent and safe medical physics practitioner or CQMP.

Certification is followed by *registration* as a CQMP, and maintenance of registration is achieved through continual professional development (CPD). Registration is effectively a formal listing of all those medical physicists who have successfully completed the certification process. In some countries this is guided by a regulatory body, while in other countries it may be done by the certifying body.

1.4.4 Recognition of the Profession

While high-income countries (HICs) have well-established systems for recognizing and supporting medical physics as a profession, there is a general lack of recognition of the profession in most LMICs. International cooperation and support are key to advancing the field and ensuring that medical physicists can effectively contribute to healthcare systems globally. To address the challenge of recognition in LMICs, the IAEA, through a series of Task Force missions, has developed a harmonized syllabus for academic and clinical training of medical physicists in an LMIC region such as Africa [17]. The syllabus spells out the roles and responsibilities, and education and training requirements for CQMPs to promote the profession globally. (Also see Chapter 11 on advocacy and diplomacy.)

1.4.5 Resource Disparities

The disparities around the globe are largely interlinked with the state of the healthcare system and available financial resources. Significant gaps exist in the availability of medical imaging and radiotherapy equipment between HICs and LMICs. LMICs can be lacking in well-educated and trained human resources, in physical resources, and in appropriate equipment for training. Furthermore, there may be limitations in terms of research capabilities for graduate students to complete their degrees.

Global medical physics considerations have been addressed in more detail by Van Dyk et al. [18]. The need for additional medical physicists is related to the ageing population globally, resulting in increased cancer incidence with approximately a 75% increase occurring in LMICs by 2030 [19], double the rate of increase compared to high-income countries (HICs). This is exacerbated by late-stage disease presentation and inaccessible diagnostics.

The following summarizes the medical physics issues, especially as related to their education and training in LMICs [18]:

- Lack of government support for appropriate healthcare-related technologies in diagnostic imaging and radiation therapy.

- Shortage of appropriate training programmes for medical physicists.

- Shortage of experienced staff to provide medical physics education and training.

- Lack of technology relevant for training medical physicists.

- Lack of appropriate recognition of medical physicists [20].

- While education abroad is often cited as an aid to the lack of education programmes, related concerns include:

  - Different diseases occur in different economic contexts; thus, the training emphasis might be different in different economic contexts.

  - LMICs have a significantly different infrastructure in both the government and educational organization, which could lead to different approaches to competencies in different economic contexts.

  - LMICs often have different treatment and diagnostic technologies compared to HICs. Thus, some of the training in an HIC context may not be relevant for LMIC contexts.

  - There is the potential for "brain drain" when students are educated in a higher-income context due to professional, economic, social, or cultural influences.

1.5 INTERNATIONAL COLLABORATION CONSIDERATIONS

There is neither single nor simple answer to solving medical physics disparities in various income environments. Multiple reports have been written on addressing these needs for radiation oncology professionals in general [21–23]. The overall theme is that there should be coordination, collaboration, and partnering between the various organizations and individuals involved in seeking support and those institutions and individuals providing support. Such support could be provided at the academic level for graduate education programmes, or at the level of clinical training in residency programmes, or in continuing education programmes. Perhaps the latter is the most common form of support from various professional organizations as well as the IAEA, in that they provide many one- to two-week short courses focused on specialized topics. The IAEA also provides support for "fellowships" which could consist of site visits for periods extending over a few months to learn about specific treatment or diagnostic procedures or quality assurance programmes or even support for graduate training over a period of two years [24].

While the demand for collaborations is substantial, there is also a significant desire for involvement in global initiatives by radiation oncology professionals. A very recent survey was designed to characterize the current levels of engagement of Canadian radiation oncologists and medical physicists in global oncology initiatives [25]. With a 79% response rate of the Canadian cancer centres from both radiation oncologists and medical physicists, 58% reported some experience with global oncology and 19% being currently directly involved in short- or long-term projects spanning 26 countries in South America, Africa, and Asia. Quality improvement and capacity building accounted for 27% and 20% of initiatives, respectively. The most common area of engagement was in direct treatment care, accounting for 56% of the projects. This is a quantitative sampling of the kind of global oncology involvement that is likely representative of the partnering that may be happening in some other countries as well.

The remaining chapters in this book address issues to consider in developing mutual benefits for international collaborations and partnerships.

1.6 SUMMARY AND RECOMMENDATIONS

1.6.1 Summary

Medical physics is a global enterprise. As the world population ages, also in LMICs, the incidence of cancers and cardiac diseases is growing dramatically. However, there are enormous variations around the world in terms of addressing the medical physics needs, especially in radiation oncology and diagnostic imaging. These relate to:

- the lack of appropriate technologies, especially for the treatment and diagnosis of cancer and cardiac patients,

- the lack of resources and infrastructure for educating and training of medical physics professionals,

- the variation in the availability and quality of education and training programmes,

- the lack of accreditation and certification of medical physics education and training programmes in different LMICs,

- the lack of professional recognition of medical physicists, especially in countries where there are only a few medical physicists.

1.6.2 Recommendations

1. Every medical physicist interested in being involved in global medical physics activities should be educated about the issues regarding global health, both from the HIC and LMIC perspectives.

2. Medical physicists interested in global health should determine where they can contribute and partner with their counterparts in other parts of the world.

3. Partnering with medical physicists in different parts of the world requires close communication between the partners, especially in understanding each other's needs. There is usually a requestor who looks for additional support, and a contributor who has the expertise to provide the additional support.

4. Involvement in global activities requires an assessment by the partners as to the sustainability of the project.

5. An educated awareness of ethical concerns regarding global collaborations is essential.

6. An educated awareness of equity, diversity, and inclusion in the context of global collaborations is essential.

7. Formal education and training for participating in global medical physics activities are essential for both those from the Global North and the Global South.

8. For those desiring to be involved in global medical physics activities, networking with professionals involved in organizations providing this type of collaboration is very helpful.

9. More detailed and in-depth information on the above recommendations can be found in subsequent chapters of this book.

REFERENCES

1. Beaglehole, R. and R. Bonita, What is global health? *Global Health Action*, 2010. **3**(1): p. 5142.
2. Castaner, X. and N. Oliveira, Collaboration, coordination, and cooperation among organizations: Establishing the distinctive meanings of these terms through a systematic literature review. *J Management*, 2020. **46**(6): p. 965–1001.
3. Wikipedia. Global north and global south. 2024 [accessed 2024-02-29]; Available from: https://en.wikipedia.org/wiki/Global_North_and_Global_South.
4. United Nations Conference on Trade and Development (UNCTAD). Country classification. 2024; Available from: https://unctadstat.unctad.org/EN/Classifications.html.
5. World Population Review. Global North. 2021; Available from: https://worldpopulationreview.com/country-rankings/global-north-countries.
6. National Geographic. Colonialism. 2024; Available from: https://www.nationalgeographic.com/culture/article/colonialism#:~:text=Colonialism%20is%20defined%20as%20%E2%80%9Ccontrol,cultural%20values%20upon%20its%20people.
7. Merriam-Webster Dictionary. Neocolonialism [accessed 2025-01-09]; Available from: https://www.merriam-webster.com/dictionary/neocolonialism.
8. Koplan, J.P., et al., Towards a common definition of global health. *Lancet*, 2009. **373**(9679): p. 1993–1995.
9. Bezak, E., J. Damilakis, and M.M. Rehani, Global status of medical physics human resource – The IOMP survey report. *Phys Med*, 2023. **113**: p. 102670.
10. Ige, T.A., et al., Medical physics development in Africa – Status, education, challenges, future. *Med Phys Int*, 2020. **8**(1): p. 303–316. http://mpijournal.org/pdf/2020-SI-03/MPI-2020-01-p303.pdf.
11. Zhu, H., et al., Global radiotherapy demands and corresponding radiotherapy-professional workforce requirements in 2022 and predicted to 2050: A population-based study. *Lancet Glob Health*, 2024. **12**(12): p. e1945–e1953.
12. Atun, R., et al., Expanding global access to radiotherapy. *Lancet Oncol*, 2015. **16**(10): p. 1153–1186.
13. Hricak, H., et al., Medical imaging and nuclear medicine: A Lancet Oncology Commission. *Lancet Oncol*, 2021. **22**(4): p. e136–e172.
14. International Atomic Energy Agency (IAEA), *Roles and Responsibilities, and Education and Training Requirements for Clinically Qualified Medical Physicists*. HHS No. 25. Human Health Series. 2013, Vienna, Austria: International Atomic Energy Agency (IAEA).
15. Chougule, A. and M. Joan, Standardization and harmonization of medical physics education and training: Survey of status. Med Phys Int J 2023. **11**(1): p. 46–49.

16. International Atomic Energy Agency (IAEA). Accreditation and certification. 2024 [accessed: 2024-02-29]; Available from: https://humanhealth .iaea.org/HHW/MedicalPhysics/TheMedicalPhysicist/EducationandTra iningRequirements/Accreditation_and_Certification/index.html#:~:text =The%20IAEA%20recommends%20that%20a%20clinically%20quali-fied%20medical,physics%20including%20radiotherapy%2C%20nuclear %20medicine%20and%20diagnostic%20radiology.

17. International Atomic Energy Agency (IAEA), Academic and clinical training programmes and portfolios for the regional training in medical physics. 2019, Vienna, Austria: International Atomic Energy Agency (IAEA) [accessed: 2024-11-26]; Available at: https://humanhealth.iaea.org/HHW /MedicalPhysics/TheMedicalPhysicist/EducationandTrainingRequire-ments/Educationalrequirements/Harmonized_syllabus_for_Medical _Physicists_training_in_Africa.pdf.

18. Van Dyk, J., D. Jaffray, and R. Jeraj, Global Considerations for the Practice of Medical Physics in Radiation Oncology, in *The Modern Technology of Radiation Oncology: A Compendium for Medical Physicists and Radiation Oncologists*, J. Van Dyk, Editor. 2020, Madison, WI: Medical Physics Publishing. p. 437–458.

19. Pramesh, C.S., *et al.*, Priorities for cancer research in low- and middle-income countries: A global perspective. *Nat Med*, 2022. **28**(4): p. 649–657.

20. Pawiro, S.A., *et al.*, Current status of medical physics recognition in SEAFOMP countries. *Med Phys Int J*, 2017. **5**(1): p. 11–15.

21. Dad, L., *et al.*, Bridging innovation and outreach to overcome global gaps in radiation oncology through information and communication tools, trainee advancement, engaging industry, attention to ethical challenges, and political advocacy. *Semin Radiat Oncol*, 2017. **27**(2): p. 98–108.

22. Ngwa, W., I. Olver, and K.M. Schmeler, The use of health-related technology to reduce the gap between developed and undeveloped regions around the globe. *Am Soc Clin Oncol Educ Book*, 2020. **40**: p. 1–10.

23. Pearlman, P.C., *et al.*, Multi-stakeholder partnerships: Breaking down barriers to effective cancer-control planning and implementation in low- and middle-income countries. *Sci Diplomacy*, 2016. **5**(1). http://www.sciencedi-plomacy.org/article/2016/multi-stakeholder-partnerships.

24. Van Dyk, J. and A. Meghzifene, The role of the International Atomic Energy Agency (IAEA) in global medical physics activities, in *Advances in Medical Physics 2014*, D.J. Godfrey, S.K. Das, and A.B. Wolbarst, Editors. 2014, Madison, WI: Medical Physics Publishing. p. 107–121.

25. Becket, M., *et al.*, Pan-Canadian survey of radiation oncology professional involvement in global oncology initiatives in low- and middle-income countries. *JCO Global Oncol*, 2024. **10**: p. e2300174.

CHAPTER 2

Challenges and Opportunities for Global Collaboration

Stephanie A. Parker and Loreh Peter Onyango

2.1 CHAPTER OBJECTIVES

- To identify how medical physicists can contribute to global collaborations in the areas of:
  - Academic medical physics education
  - Clinical medical physics training
  - Global research and scientific innovation
- To explain how structure and support are provided to global collaborations through:
  - Needs assessments
  - Liaison networks
  - Data and information exchange
- To discuss best practices and potential challenges in global medical physics collaborations
- To provide recommendations on challenges and opportunities for global collaborations of medical physicists

DOI: 10.1201/9781003527749-2

2.2 INTRODUCTION TO GLOBAL COLLABORATIONS

Global collaborations in medical physics vary with respect to scale and scope. Collaborations occur between individuals, institutions, organizations, or governments, and are bilateral (involving two parties) or multilateral (involving more than two). Global collaborations may range from small-scale, short-term projects to long-term, large-scale inter-institutional initiatives. The key to a successful collaboration is mutual benefit among all parties and a common long-term goal of improving health.

To ensure that global collaborations are effective, certain characteristics should be present: clear goals, a well-defined scope, specific outcomes, established processes to achieve these outcomes, as well as project closeout and follow-up. For long-term collaborations, setting intermediate goals or identifying a series of shorter-term projects provides structure and maintains momentum. If a collaborative project is of large scale, conducting small-scale pilot projects can test feasibility and establish best practices. Pilot projects should be designed with scalability in mind to prevent "pilotitis," which occurs when multiple small-scale projects are conducted without a scale-up plan [1].

Various models of global health collaborations have been proposed. In the context of academic medicine and global health, Sewankambo proposed a four-prong approach: research, evidence-based implementation, education, and service delivery [2]. The World Health Organization's (WHO) Global Health and Peace Initiative outlines six "workstreams" that guide collaborations: research, framework development, advocacy, capacity-building, developing partnerships, and mainstreaming (i.e., implementation) [3]. The American Association of Physicists in Medicine (AAPM) established an International Council in 2021 with a structure consisting of needs assessment, education, clinical training, research, information exchange, and global liaisons. Medical physics global collaborations typically focus on research and innovation, academic education, or clinical training. Needs assessment, liaison development, and information management provide structure and foster knowledge sharing and, therefore, should encompass all collaborative projects (see Figure 2.1). The following sections will discuss each element of the AAPM's structure for global collaboration.

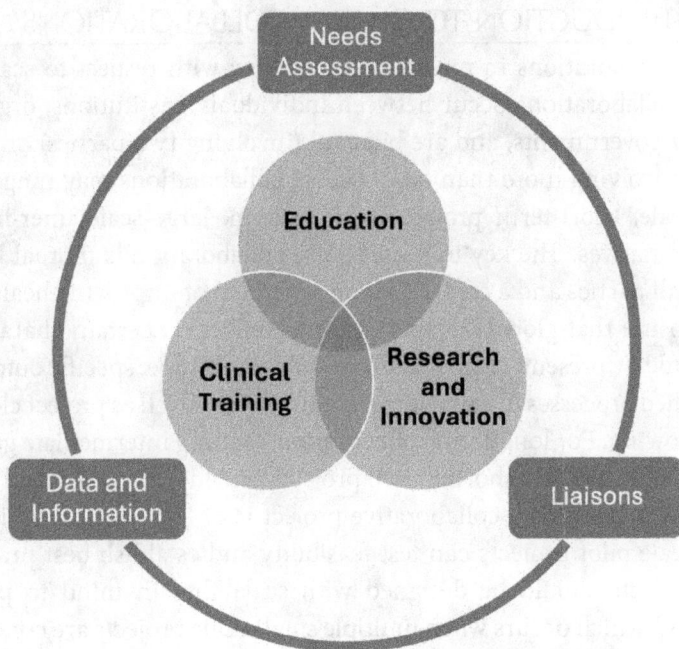

FIGURE 2.1 Needs assessment, liaisons, and data and information provide structure and support for global medical physics collaborations in the areas of education, clinical training, and research and innovation.

2.3 GLOBAL NEEDS ASSESSMENT

A needs assessment is a prospective, systematic process for identifying and prioritizing needs. The purpose of a global health needs assessment is to collect information that will drive change to improve population health. The scope can vary widely and include assessment of needs for individuals, groups, populations, institutions, organizations, or regions.

Needs can be classified into normative, felt, expressed, and comparative [4]. Normative need is measured relative to a standard. For example, the number of linear accelerators in a country can be compared to the International Atomic Energy Agency (IAEA) recommended number based on population. Felt need is based on individual perceptions, such as a low- and middle-income country (LMIC) medical physicist identifying a need for additional equipment. Expressed need is an action taken to request goods or services, such as an LMIC medical physicist requesting equipment donations. Comparative needs are needs identified by comparing resources between different individuals, groups, locations, etc. An example would be identifying the need for linear accelerators in an LMIC based on the relative number of linear accelerators between the LMIC and high-income countries (HICs).

Healthcare needs assessments include approaches involving corporate, community, comparative, and epidemiological frameworks. Corporate approaches involve gathering information from local health professionals and patients [5], while community approaches gather information from community members as healthcare consumers [6]. Both approaches provide insight into local practices and help garner local support for collaborative projects. Comparative approaches assess the differences in services and outcomes between two populations [5], while epidemiological approaches analyze population and health data such as incidence of disease and use of health services [5, 7]. Both comparative and epidemiological approaches can identify gaps in healthcare needs for a population. Additionally, these two approaches may be combined through a comparison of epidemiological data between populations or over time for the same population.

Methods of needs assessments include interviews, inventories, direct observation, focus group discussions, surveys, data searches, and combinations of methods (mixed methods). Each method has advantages and limitations. Interviews, inventories, and focus groups are time-consuming and typically involve small groups; surveys and data analyses are better suited for large populations but can suffer from sampling bias. Mixed methods allow the ability to validate and triangulate data. Combining qualitative and quantitative methods can provide a deeper assessment of the needs of a population or region. For example, qualitative surveys can provide an overview of medical physicists' needs in a global region, while structured interviews can offer detailed insight into specific challenges.

The goal of a needs assessment is to identify needs that can be addressed through action. Once data is analyzed and needs identified, they should be prioritized with input from all stakeholders. Prioritization can involve both quantitative and qualitative approaches. Quantitative methods include identifying the greatest needs from surveys or identifying the most prevalent stage at diagnosis for cancer types in a global region. Such information can allow the prioritization of resources such as which cancer screening programmes to implement first. Qualitative methods may involve the ranking of the importance of needs by local healthcare workers or the identification of projects with a high probability of success that will build trust and establish relationships before tackling larger, more complex projects.

Once needs are prioritized, the information should be disseminated to those responsible for addressing them such as global partners and organizations. Throughout the process, progress should be monitored, and upon project completion, feedback should be collected and analyzed. Identifying best practices and lessons learned will enhance future collaborations. As needs assessments represent only a snapshot in time, they should be conducted periodically to track progress and adjust priorities.

See Figure 2.2 for a general global needs assessment process.

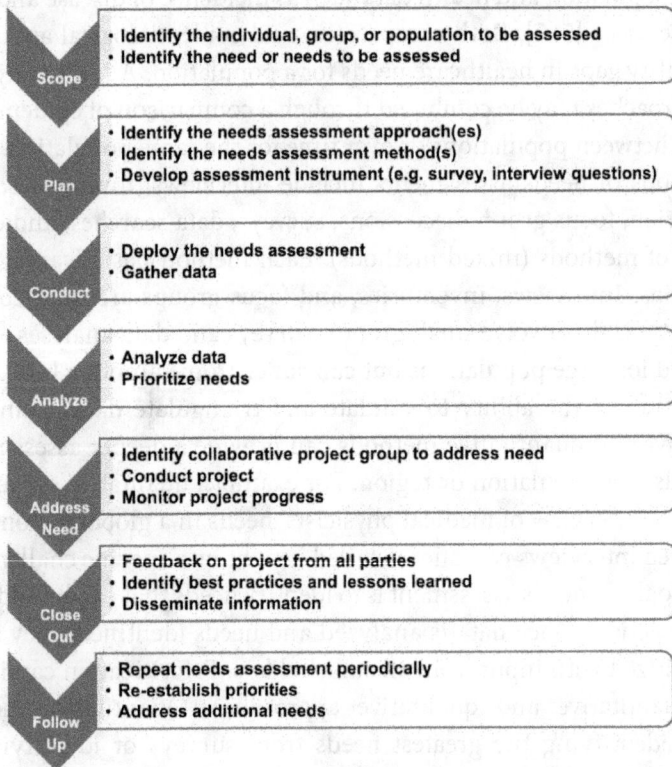

Scope
- Identify the individual, group, or population to be assessed
- Identify the need or needs to be assessed

Plan
- Identify the needs assessment approach(es)
- Identify the needs assessment method(s)
- Develop assessment instrument (e.g. survey, interview questions)

Conduct
- Deploy the needs assessment
- Gather data

Analyze
- Analyze data
- Prioritize needs

Address Need
- Identify collaborative project group to address need
- Conduct project
- Monitor project progress

Close Out
- Feedback on project from all parties
- Identify best practices and lessons learned
- Disseminate information

Follow Up
- Repeat needs assessment periodically
- Re-establish priorities
- Address additional needs

FIGURE 2.2 A general needs assessment process includes identifying the scope, developing a plan, conducting the needs assessment, analyzing the data, addressing the need through a collaborative project, project closeout, and follow-up.

2.4 DEVELOPING GLOBAL LIAISONS

Many groups and organizations participate in global medical physics activities. However, suboptimal communication between these groups can lead to duplication of effort and silos of knowledge. Experience gained by one group should be shared, preventing lessons from being learned repeatedly. Partnering allows groups to leverage strengths. Global health resources are limited, and duplicating effort is inefficient. Establishing a network of global liaisons can combat silos, reduce effort duplication, and identify opportunities for collaboration.

The first step in establishing a global liaison network is to identify the key players in global medical physics, radiology, and radiation oncology. Once these groups or organizations are identified, a point of contact should be established. An analysis or inventory of each group should be conducted to include the areas of focus, scope of activities, and expected role in global health initiatives. Additionally, it is important to be aware of organizational mandates that limit activities and memoranda of understanding (MOUs) between organizations.

The next step is to identify what global collaborations have occurred in the past, which are in progress, and what is being planned. Are there prior experiences – both positive and negative – that can be leveraged? Is there overlap between collaborations that can be streamlined? Do the organizations have experience in specific global regions? Are there organizations with expertise in scaling up solutions? Collecting this information will provide a comprehensive overview of global health activities in medical physics and related fields, reveal gaps in the global landscape, and identify the optimal stakeholders for future collaborations.

When establishing global collaborations, an important liaison will be the end users of the collaboration's product(s). End users may range from individual health professionals or hospitals to countries or entire global regions, and the collaboration's goals should align with their needs and expectations.

2.5 GLOBAL DATA AND INFORMATION EXCHANGE

Information is the scaffold that supports and connects all global health activities. Data should drive global efforts, with information shared rather than isolated. The success of the collaborations hinges on effective information management. Not only does it support individual collaborations, but also helps create a comprehensive database of projects that can be leveraged for a broader impact. Data should guide the prioritization of collaborations and the identification of best practices. As discussed previously, siloed activities waste resources and can have detrimental effects on global health. Sharing information is essential to breaking down silos and ensuring efficient use of resources for maximum benefit. Chapter 13 provides further details on global collaboration on data sharing.

2.6 GLOBAL RESEARCH AND SCIENTIFIC INNOVATION

Research provides valuable insight into health challenges. Although LMICs shoulder the majority of global disease burden, most research is conducted in HICs [8]. Research in HICs may not directly translate to LMICs for several reasons.

- Health challenges and diseases most prevalent in HICs differ from those in LMICs.

- Biomedical solutions developed in HICs may not be feasible in LMICs due to differences in infrastructure, resources, technology, and sustainability.

- Translation and implementation frameworks developed in HICs to move research into action may not be compatible with the healthcare systems and cultural contexts of LMICs.

Given these challenges, research should be conducted in LMICs, ideally led by or in collaboration with local researchers.

Research also presents an opportunity to enhance staff retention and mitigate "brain drain." A survey of medical physicists found that over half enjoyed conducting research, even inspiring many to remain in the field [9]. Thus, research opportunities have the potential to increase and retain the medical physics workforce in LMICs. Collaborations with medical physicists in both HICs and other LMICs can empower LMIC medical physicist researchers. Developing innovative solutions to radiation therapy, radiology, and medical physics challenges specific to LMICs is an area of great promise. However, LMIC scientists often face difficulties establishing research careers due to underrepresentation in peer-reviewed publications and scientific conferences – both critical avenues for professional visibility and securing funding. Chapter 3 addresses the benefits and challenges of global collaborations.

2.7 GLOBAL MEDICAL PHYSICS EDUCATION

To become Clinically Qualified Medical Physicists (CQMPs), individuals must either obtain a postgraduate degree in medical physics or in a related field coupled with relevant medical physics coursework [10]. While medical physics education programmes are vital for increasing the number of professionals in LMICs, these programmes are limited in number. Ige et al. report that only eight African countries offer medical physics graduate programmes [11]. Furthermore, a survey of radiology and radiation therapy institutions in LMICs found that only 34% of respondents were affiliated with formal medical physics education programmes [12].

Establishing medical physics graduate programmes in LMICs requires significant institutional support and faculty time for curriculum development and instruction. Global collaborations should prioritize educating medical physicists in their home countries, in environments similar to those in which they will practice.

Collaborations between HIC and LMIC institutions can help expand the number and capacity of medical physics programmes in LMICs. Bilateral or multilateral partnerships between educational institutions could allow students to attend lectures remotely and faculty to share teaching responsibilities. HIC institutions could also grant access to libraries and reference materials for LMIC students. A challenge in establishing educational programmes is the cost of medical physics equipment [13]. Professional organizations could donate equipment to reduce this burden. As with all collaborations, it is essential that each party plays an active role in setting the agenda.

2.8 GLOBAL MEDICAL PHYSICS CLINICAL TRAINING

Clinical training encompasses both training as part of the initial educational process such as residencies and training for new clinical procedures and equipment. Clinical training spans medical physics careers as the field evolves and new techniques introduced.

Structured clinical training of no less than two years is required for medical physicists to become Clinically Qualified Medical Physicists (CQMPs) [10]. Collaborations can assist LMICs in the clinical training of medical physicists. Establishing residency programmes necessitates designing curricula that include appropriate rotations, creating syllabi for each rotation, developing assessments, and setting competency criteria. This is a substantial undertaking and is often completed ad hoc around clinical responsibilities. Collaboration in the form of twinning – between an established residency programme (in an HIC or LMIC) and a new programme in an LMIC – could enable the LMIC residency programme director to leverage the experience of the established programme's director, utilizing their curricula and assessments as a foundation. Forming multilateral partnerships (consortia) among multiple residency programmes could facilitate resource sharing and distribute the administrative burden. If specific procedures or equipment are not available at all institutions, residents could temporarily travel to other training sites to gain the necessary experience. However, challenges associated with these collaborations may include the need to formalize relationships between institutions, which can be difficult in securing buy-in and support from leadership. Additionally, the institutions must have compatible clinical programmes to collaborate effectively, and the expense of travel to other locations for specific procedure training may also pose a challenge.

Medical physics is a constantly evolving field with new procedures and techniques introduced continuously. Practicing medical physicists must be trained and develop competency in new techniques before clinical implementation. Training and programme development can be supported through global collaborations at the peer, institutional, and organizational levels. Peer-level collaborations have proven beneficial in the implementation of techniques such as IMRT [14]. Institutional collaborations have been useful in developing programmes such as SBRT [15] and new technology such as automated treatment planning [16]. As with other collaborations, it is crucial to ensure that processes are adapted to the resources available in LMICs and that medical physicists from these countries are actively and equitably involved. While virtual training can partially fulfil clinical training requirements, in-person training in the environment where the procedures will be performed, using the actual equipment, remains a necessary component.

2.9 SUMMARY AND RECOMMENDATIONS

2.9.1 Summary
Global medical physics collaborations have the potential to address healthcare challenges in LMICs and build capacity in the areas of education,

clinical training, and research. Needs assessments, global liaisons, and information management guide and support these efforts. All collaborations should include LMIC medical physicists and institutions when setting the agenda. Regardless of type or scale, the key to a successful collaboration is mutual benefit among all parties.

2.9.2 Recommendations

1. Global collaborations should include clear goals, a well-defined scope, desired outcomes, established processes, closeout, and follow-up.

2. Pilot projects should be designed with scalability in mind to prevent "pilotitis."

3. Needs assessments should use data to identify needs that can be addressed through action.

4. Prioritization of collaborative projects should involve input from all stakeholders.

5. A network of global liaisons should be established to provide collective knowledge and experience that can be leveraged during global collaborations.

6. Organizations engaged in global health activities should develop clear data policies.

7. Global medical physics research collaborations should prioritize building research capacity in LMICs, co-establishing the research agenda with LMIC physicists, fostering long-term collaborative relationships, and ensuring LMIC authorship on publications.

8. Global education collaborations should focus on educating medical physicists in their home countries and in a similar environment that they will practice upon graduating.

9. Global clinical training collaborations at the residency level should be developed to facilitate resource sharing and distribute the administrative burden.

10. While virtual training can partially fulfil clinical training requirements, in-person training in the environment where the procedures will be performed, using the actual equipment, remains a necessary component.

REFERENCES

1. Huang, F., S. Blaschke, and H. Lucas, Beyond pilotitis: Taking digital health interventions to the national level in China and Uganda. *Globalization and Health*, 2017. **13**(1): p. 49.
2. Sewankambo, N., Academic medicine and global health responsibilities. *BMJ*, 2004. **329**(7469): p. 752–753.
3. World Health Organization. WHO Global Health and Peace Initiative (GHPI). 2024 [cited 2024 October 29]; Available from: https://www.who.int/initiatives/who-health-and-peace-initiative.
4. Bradshaw, J., A Taxonomy of social need, in *Problems and Progress in Medical Care: Essays on Current Research*, G. McLachlan, Editor. 1972, Oxford University Press: London.
5. Stevens, A., and S. Gillam, Needs assessment: From theory to practice. *BMJ*, 1998. **316**(7142): p. 1448–1452.
6. Wright, J., and J. Walley, Assessing health needs in developing countries. *BMJ*, 1998. **316**(7147): p. 1819–1823.
7. Wright, J., R. Williams, and J.R. Wilkinson, Development and importance of health needs assessment. *BMJ*, 1998. **316**(7140): p. 1310–1313.
8. Langer, A., C. Díaz-Olavarrieta, K. Berdichevsky, *et al.*, Why is research from developing countries underrepresented in international health literature, and what can be done about it? *Bulletin of the World Health Organization*, 2004. **82**(10): p. 802–803.
9. Ebert, M.A., G.K.B. Halkett, M. Berg, *et al.*, An assessment of radiation oncology medical physicists' perspectives on undertaking research. *Australasian Physical & Engineering Sciences in Medicine*, 2017. **40**(1): p. 173–180.
10. International Atomic Energy Agency, Roles and responsibilities, and education and training requirements for clinically qualified medical physicists, in *IAEA Human Health Series*. 2013, International Atomic Energy Agency: Vienna.
11. Ige, T.A., Hasford, F., Tabakov, S., *et al.*, Medical physics development in Africa: Status, education, challenges, future. *Medical Physics International*, **2020**(3): p. 303–316.
12. Parker, S., J. Weygand, B. Bernat, *et al.*, Assessing radiology and radiotherapy needs for cancer care in low-and-middle-income countries: Insights from a global survey of departmental and institutional leaders. *Advances in Radiation Oncology*, 2024. **9**: p. 101615.
13. Bezak, E., J. Damilakis, and M.M. Rehani, Global status of medical physics human resource – The IOMP survey report. *Physica Medica*, 2023. **113**: p. 102670.

14. Mohamad, I., A. Salem, T. Abu Hejleh, *et al.*, Peer-assisted learning: Intensity-modulated radiotherapy transition in developing countries. *Clinical Oncology*, 2017. **29**(10): p. 689–695.
15. Khader, J., A. Al-Mousa, F.A. Hijla, *et al.*, Requirements and implementation of a lung SBRT program in a developing country: Benefits of international cooperation. *Int J Radiat Oncol Biol Phys*, 2016. **95**(4): p. 1236–8.
16. Trauernicht, C., and L. Court, The value of global collaborations. *Journal of Applied Clinical Medical Physics*, 2024. **25**(4): p. e14334.

CHAPTER 3

Building Global Inter-Institutional Collaborations

Dario Sanz, Martin Ebert,
Mauro Namias, and Robert Jeraj

3.1 CHAPTER OBJECTIVES

- To characterize different types of global collaborations, with an emphasis on inter-institutional collaborations

- To describe how global collaborations can be developed and be of benefit

- To describe challenges associated with global collaborations

  - Administrative challenges

  - Clinical challenges

  - Infrastructural and technical challenges

- To address ethical issues in global collaborations

- To provide recommendations on building global medical physics collaborations

DOI: 10.1201/9781003527749-3

3.2 INTRODUCTION

Collaboration is the process of individuals, groups of people, or organizations working together to achieve a planned goal. It includes the sharing of ideas, knowledge, resources, and responsibilities, and requires effective communication, coordination, deadlines, and mutual respect among participants. Successful collaboration often generates advanced solutions, improved efficiency, and better outcomes than could be achieved individually. It can exist in various contexts including scientific, academic, professional, social, and creative environments.

In an era where healthcare demands are increasingly complex and resources are often stretched thin, collaboration has emerged as a strategic approach to enhance the efficiency, effectiveness, and quality of patient care. For healthcare centres such as hospitals and clinics, engaging in collaborative programmes with other individuals, healthcare, or research centres can offer numerous benefits. These benefits include shared resources, improved access to specialized expertise, and enhanced innovation. However, the success of such collaborations hinges critically on a comprehensive understanding of the unique challenges each collaborator faces. This understanding is not merely beneficial but fundamental to optimizing the collaboration and achieving its full potential.

While collaboration in health-related activities can range from simple interactions between two individuals to complex international, multi-institutional efforts, this chapter focuses on inter-institutional collaborations. Healthcare is often provided by large institutions, especially in areas involving medical physicists, such as radiation therapy, imaging, nuclear medicine, research and academic areas, among others. We also detail inter-professional, intra-institutional collaborations, which are crucial for the success of inter-institutional efforts. Successful inter-institutional collaboration is unlikely if there are failures within intra-institutional collaborations.

Identifying and acknowledging challenges within each institution allow for the creation of tailored strategies that address specific issues, thereby enhancing the overall efficacy of the collaboration. For instance, hospitals struggling with outdated technologies will emphasize technology upgrades and training; however, hospitals with staff shortages will direct efforts towards joint recruitment or encouraging education programmes.

Transparency about challenges fosters trust and open communication between collaborating entities. When institutions are upfront with their difficulties, it sets a precedent for honesty and mutual support, encouraging sustainability of the partnership.

3.3 FOSTERING EFFECTIVE COLLABORATION AND EVIDENCE OF SUCCESS

Exploring this complex area of organizational behaviour can be both challenging and rewarding. Research indicates that fostering collaborative practice requires providing physical and structural opportunities, creating a psychologically supportive environment, and offering adequate education and training. Evidence has emerged for positive outcomes from fostered collaboration.

Effective intra-institutional collaboration is critically based on inter-professional collaboration within the institution. Inter-professional collaboration is critical to a well-functioning healthcare team that ensures high quality and safe patient care, enhances satisfaction and engagement among both patients and staff, and promotes organizational efficiency and innovation [1]. Effective collaboration in healthcare teams is influenced by a variety of factors, including the dynamics of interpersonal relationships within the team (*interactional determinants*), conditions within the organization (*organizational determinants*), and the organization environment (*systemic determinants*) [2].

Key elements for successful collaboration include establishing clear organizational structures, such as common rules and effective information systems, and ensuring that professionals have the time, space, and resources to interact and address issues. Promoting inter-professional collaboration is not solely the responsibility of managers and policymakers; it also requires active participation from professionals themselves [3].

Inter-professional teams encompass all areas that contribute to healthcare, either directly or indirectly, including teaching and research teams, healthcare professionals (e.g., medical physicists, engineers, technicians, computer specialists, doctors), administrative staff, and authorities. These team members often come from different institutions, e.g., teaching and research professionals may be affiliated with a university, while others work at a hospital. This naturally leads to inter-institutional collaboration.

It is widely accepted that team size and diversity facilitate scientific developments [4]. Such progress must be supported by effective collaborations. The link between research, innovation, and clinical practice is sustainable only through robust inter-institutional partnerships and global collaborations [1, 5, 6].

In clinical practice, particularly in medical physics, collaboration is multifaceted and occurs at multiple levels. It involves various forms of engagement, including cooperation agreements, transnational research organizations, funding programmes, international scientific exchanges, open access publishing, consumer engagement, and scientific advisory committees to governing bodies. Examples of successful intra-institutional collaboration in the medical physics context include establishing medical physics education and training programmes in low- to middle-income countries (LMICs), recognition of medical physics as a healthcare profession, and training of medical physicists in reference centres [7].

The distinctions between research and clinical service significantly influence how international collaborations are structured and managed. Research collaborations are typically more flexible and exploratory, focusing on innovation and knowledge generation, while clinical service collaborations prioritize safety, consistency, and the immediate application of established medical practices.

3.4 COLLABORATION CHALLENGES

Inter-institutional collaboration programmes can face significant challenges. The main difficulties arise from team dynamics, such as when members act as representatives of their professions rather than as a cohesive unit [8]. Other issues include the interaction of diverse knowledge contributions and the influence of the surrounding organization. These challenges can limit the effective use of collaborative resources.

Understanding the differences between different focus areas (e.g., diagnostics vs therapy) is essential for designing and managing successful international collaborations. These differences impact team composition, regulatory compliance, data management, training, and research focus.

It's important to distinguish these collaborative challenges from the initial problems that necessitated the collaboration, which can be administrative, clinical, or infrastructural. These will be detailed in the following section. Before initiating or expanding collaborations, it is highly advisable to perform a SWOT (Strengths, Weaknesses, Opportunities, Threats) analysis within the environment involved. An insightful editorial [9] suggests asking, "What should we start doing?" "What should we stop doing?" and "What should we keep doing?" It also emphasizes protecting past gains amid changes.

To ensure that professionals can fulfil their roles and responsibilities effectively, administrative, clinical, and infrastructural challenges must be minimal or actively managed. For instance, addressing the shortage of clinically qualified medical physicists, the need for education and training, and enhancing professional recognition are critical steps identified for clinical improvement [10].

The importance of well-structured goals and milestones with clear deadlines is critical for any successful collaboration. A well-thought-out and realistic timeline, which outlines the duration and phases of the collaboration, plays a pivotal role in ensuring that the partnership achieves its objectives. This timeline should be viewed as a function of several inherent variables, including the specific challenges each institution faces, the resources available, and the milestones that need to be met for the collaboration to be successful.

3.5 CHALLENGES NECESSITATING COLLABORATION

Understanding each institution's challenges enables better resource allocation. Resources can be distributed more effectively when there is a clear picture of where they are needed most. This approach prevents wastage and ensures that critical issues are addressed promptly, thereby maximizing the impact of the collaboration.

Acknowledging and addressing existing problems can serve as a baseline for measuring the success of the collaboration. By setting clear benchmarks based on initial challenges, institutions can track progress and make data-driven decisions to refine and improve collaborative efforts over time. To address the problems and challenges commonly encountered in clinics, one must examine administrative and management issues, clinical and patient care problems, and infrastructural and technological challenges.

Hospitals often share facilities with university and research laboratories or have formal agreements with academic institutions and research groups. Smaller clinics may establish partnerships with research centres for human resource education or technological and procedural innovations. Industrial collaborations potentially involve legal agreements and aggressive timelines. Consequently, analyzing the challenges faced by collaborating institutions inherently includes those related to academic and research areas, as they are integral to the healthcare environment.

3.6 ADMINISTRATIVE AND MANAGEMENT CHALLENGES

3.6.1 Human Resources

The human resource component is critical. The number and expertise of staff should align with the relevant demands. However, financial constraints often result in staffing levels that are suboptimal. Furthermore, inadequate training or expertise can exacerbate this situation. Additional challenges include high staff turnover, insufficient full-time staff, and a lack of support staff.

While funding is a significant factor, other elements such as institutional procedures and organizational practices also impact on the balance of staff numbers and their quality. Addressing these issues requires a comprehensive approach that goes beyond financial considerations to include strategic improvements in management and policy.

3.6.2 Procedures and Organization

Effective procedures and robust organizational structures are vital for maintaining a high standard of healthcare services. However, several factors can undermine this goal. The absence of educational programmes, continuing education, and training hampers staff development, preventing healthcare professionals from staying updated with the latest practices and technologies. Additionally, lack of accreditation, certification, and registration further exacerbates the issue by failing to ensure that staff meet the required standards of proficiency and competency [10].

Inadequate human resource development results in a workforce that is not fully prepared to meet the demands of their roles, with insufficient opportunities for professional growth and skill enhancement. Poor organizational structures within institutions contribute to inefficiencies and a lack of coordination, often resulting in overlapping responsibilities and unclear job roles. Insufficient support from health authorities, who may prioritize other healthcare areas, leaves gaps in essential services and support for staff.

Unfortunately, and as a significant challenge, qualified staff may be reluctant to share specific knowledge or teach other, leading to knowledge silos and preventing the dissemination of critical information and best practices. Additionally, staff often juggle multiple responsibilities, including teaching and administrative tasks, detracting from their ability to focus on specific job functions. Poor working conditions, including the excessive effort required for quality assurance tasks, contribute to job dissatisfaction and burnout.

Ineffective communication among staff hinders knowledge transfer and collaboration, resulting in missed opportunities for improvement and innovation. High levels of job stress affect staff well-being and performance, leading to decreased productivity and increased errors. There is also a lack of motivation, opportunity, and funding for staff to present their work at conferences, which is essential for demonstrating competencies and fostering professional growth. Limited access to current literature and resources further stifles development.

3.7 CLINICAL AND PATIENT CARE CHALLENGES

Ensuring high-quality care in healthcare settings, particularly in radiological services, involves addressing several critical issues. A primary concern is the lack of radiation safety and protection for patients, staff, and the general public in LMICs. This issue is compounded by the absence of regulatory bodies or deficiencies in regulation and enforcement. When regulatory frameworks are weak or inspections are ineffective, compliance with safety standards becomes inconsistent.

Non-compliance with regulations or a lack of enforcement power further undermines safety protocols. This often results in the inadequate implementation of a quality assurance (QA) programme, such as proper documentation, especially for incidents like radiological mishaps. Proper documentation is essential for developing and updating institutional policies and procedures related to radiation use.

Another significant issue is the reluctance to accept external collaborations, such as audits, expert visits, or intercomparison events. This refusal or lack of transparency in working methods can be perceived as a threat to quality, as it hinders objective assessment and potential improvements. Open collaboration is thus crucial for identifying gaps and implementing best practices.

3.8 INDUSTRIAL COLLABORATIONS

Industrial collaborations have their own unique considerations, including issues related to research and development, clinical and applications training for the use of new technologies, in addition to participating in clinical trials. Because of financial motivations, ethical issues need careful consideration. Note that Chapter 5 is fully devoted to addressing global collaborations with industry.

3.9 INFRASTRUCTURAL AND TECHNOLOGICAL CHALLENGES

The quality and effectiveness of healthcare services are heavily influenced by the state of physical infrastructure. One of the primary challenges is insufficient funding, which leads to a cascade of related issues. The lack and deficiency of technical maintenance staff results in deteriorating facilities and equipment. This is further exacerbated by an insufficient amount of equipment and technology needed for treatment and diagnosis, particularly in LMICs where such technology is typically imported. Furthermore, the unavailability of spare parts, coupled with the obsolescence or frequent failure of existing equipment, hampers the ability to provide consistent and reliable care. Failures in utilities, such as unstable electricity supply, also disrupt healthcare operations, while a lack of physical space or functional limitations, along with poor building maintenance and the inability to expand spatially, further constrain service delivery.

Innovation and technological adaptation are also critical areas of concern. There is often a failure to fully utilize the technological capabilities of existing equipment due to a lack of knowledge, necessary accessories, proper authorizations, clinical disinterest, or insufficient promotion. Also, resistance to new technologies and methods, and the prevalence of a conservative structure, delay progress, and adaptation. Additionally, the absence of necessary ancillary or diagnostic services, such as PET or MRI for a radiotherapy service or diagnosis, limits the ability to offer comprehensive and high-quality clinical care.

All the abovementioned issues should be described and quantified as a necessary condition before entering a particular collaboration.

3.10 ETHICS IN GLOBAL COLLABORATIONS

Ethics plays a fundamental role in the success and integrity of global collaborations in healthcare. Ethical considerations ensure that the partnerships are not only effective but also equitable and just [11–14]. In addition to the conventional overarching ethical pillars of beneficence, non-maleficence, autonomy, and justice, some key ethical and governance principles that should guide inter-institutional collaborations include:

- Transparency and honesty
- Equity and fairness

- Respect for autonomy
- Clarity around ownership
- Confidentiality
- Accountability
- Cultural sensitivity
- Sustainability

By embedding these ethical principles into the framework of global collaborations, healthcare institutions can ensure that their partnerships are not only effective but also just and equitable, ultimately leading to better health outcomes and stronger, more resilient healthcare systems worldwide. Note that Chapter 15 is fully devoted to ethical considerations in global collaborations.

3.11 SUMMARY AND RECOMMENDATIONS

3.11.1 Summary

Inter-institutional collaboration in healthcare is crucial for improving efficiency, effectiveness, and the quality of patient care, especially given the complex and resource-strained nature of modern healthcare demands. Such collaborations offer benefits like shared resources, specialized expertise, and enhanced innovation. However, their success relies on understanding and addressing the unique challenges each participating institution faces.

Identifying these challenges allows for tailored strategies, improving the collaboration's efficacy. Transparency about these challenges fosters trust and open communication, essential for sustainable partnerships. Trust ensures that all parties are invested in finding solutions and sharing the risks and rewards.

Effective collaboration requires clear organizational structures, physical and structural opportunities, and a supportive environment. Key factors influencing successful collaboration include interpersonal dynamics, organizational conditions, and systemic determinants. Collaboration should involve all stakeholders, including healthcare professionals, teaching and research staff, and administrative authorities.

However, collaborations can face significant challenges, such as team dynamics, diverse knowledge contributions, and organizational influences. Addressing these requires a thorough understanding of administrative, clinical, and infrastructural challenges.

3.11.2 Recommendations

1. **Determine Collaboration Goals**: Begin by identifying and prioritizing the challenges that should be addressed. Conduct a SWOT analysis. Outline specific goals, with clear milestones and timelines.

2. **Identify Resource Constraints**: Predict necessary resources that are available, and will continue to be available, while also considering day-to-day constraints of the inter-institutional collaborative teams.

3. **Determine the Main Collaboration Challenges**: Some of the most important challenges are listed below:

   a. **Enhance Procedures and Organizational Structures**:

      i. Use robust educational programmes and continuous education initiatives.

      ii. Ensure proper accreditation, certification, and registration procedures for all staff members.

      iii. Foster a culture of knowledge sharing and professional growth.

   b. **Address Human Resource Development**:

      i. Encourage qualified staff to share their knowledge, teach others, and foster mentorship.

      ii. Manage workloads effectively.

      iii. Encourage staff to present their work both at home and at conferences.

      iv. Stay abreast of the current literature.

   c. **Ensure Quality of Care**:

      i. Enforce robust regulatory frameworks to ensure the safety of patient care.

      ii. Promote transparency and encourage external collaborations, such as audits.

      iii. Adequate service coverage is essential to prevent gaps in care.

      iv. Continuous improvement in safety practices should be a priority to protect both patients and staff.

   d. **Improve Developments in Infrastructure and Equipment**:

      i. Secure adequate funding for the maintenance and acquisition of new equipment.

    ii. Ensure the availability of accessory equipment and spare parts.

    iii. Address urban service failures as feasible within the circumstances.

e. **Explore Technological Innovation**:

    i. Collaborations could include enhanced utilization of existing equipment capabilities and overcoming resistance to new technologies and methods.

    ii. Ensure the availability or improvement of diagnostic services.

    iii. Develop a robust system for regular equipment maintenance.

    iv. Develop a system for staff training to handle advanced equipment and new techniques.

f. **Incorporate Ethical Aspects of Collaborations**:

    i. Uphold strong ethical standards to foster effective and equitable partnerships.

g. **Foster an Environment of Transparency and Honesty**:

    i. Openly share strengths, weaknesses, and resource needs.

    ii. Disclose potential conflicts of interest.

    iii. Equity and fairness must be central to the collaboration, ensuring an equal voice and access to resources, including a fair distribution of the benefits of the collaboration.

    iv. Respect each institution's autonomy.

h. **Protect Confidentiality**:

    i. Of sensitive information, such as patient data and proprietary research.

    ii. Regular monitoring, evaluation, and transparent reporting of progress are crucial for accountability.

    iii. Address issues and challenges promptly.

i. **Uphold Cultural Sensitivity**:

    i. Ensure that the partnership is inclusive and respectful of all participants.

REFERENCES

1. Lyndon Morley, and Angela Cashell 2017, Continuing medical education collaboration in health care. *Journal of Medical Imaging and Radiation Sciences.* 48(2): 207–216.
2. San Martin-Rodriguez M. et al. 2005, The determinants of successful collaboration: A review of theoretical and empirical studies. *Journal of Interprofessional Care.* 19(Suppl 1): 132–147.
3. Evert Schota, Lars Tummersa, and Mirko Noordegraaf 2020, Working on working together. A systematic review on how healthcare professionals contribute to interprofessional collaboration. *Journal of Interprofessional Care.* 34(3): 332–342.
4. Wuchty S, Jones BF, Uzzi B 2007, The increasing dominance of teams in production of knowledge. *Science.* 2316(5827):1036–1039. doi: 10.1126/science.1136099.
5. Chris Trauernicht, Laurence Court 2024, The value of global collaborations. *Journal of Applied Clinical Medical Physics.* 25(4):e14334.
6. Manjit Dosanjh 2022, Collaboration: The Force that makes the impossible possible. *Advances in Radiation Oncology.* 7(6):100966.
7. Tabakov S, Stoeva M. 2021, Collaborative networking and support for medical physics development in low and middle income (LMI) countries. Health Technology (Berlin). 11(5):963–969.
8. Kvarnström, S. 2008, Difficulties in collaboration: A critical incident study of interprofessional healthcare teamwork. *Journal of Interprofessional Care.* 22(2): 191–203.
9. Jordan D, Gingold E, Samei E 2019, Editorial: Automation, regulation, and collaboration: Threats and opportunities for clinical medical physics careers in diagnostic imaging and nuclear medicine. *Journal of Applied Clinical Medical Physics.* 20(5):4–6.
10. International Atomic Energy Agency (IAEA) 2013, *Roles and Responsibilities, Education and Training Requirements for Clinically Qualified Medical Physicists*, IAEA Human Health Series No. 25, International Atomic Energy Agency, Vienna.
11. American Association of Physicists in Medicine 2019, *Code of Ethics for the American Association of Physicists in Medicine (Revised): Report of Task Group 109.* Available at: https://aapm.onlinelibrary.wiley.com/doi/10.1002/mp.13351 [Accessed 2025-02-01]
12. American Association of Physicists in Medicine 2010, *Code Recommended Ethics Curriculum for Medical Physics Graduate and Residency Programs*, Rep. No. 159, AAPM, College Park, MD. Available at: https://aapm.onlinelibrary.wiley.com/doi/10.1118/1.3451116. [Accessed 2024-11-21]
13. International Atomic Energy Agency (IAEA) 2023, *Guidelines on Professional Ethics for Medical Physicists, TCS 78.* International Atomic Energy Agency (IAEA): Vienna, Austria.
14. Health and Care Professions Council 2012, Standards of conduct, performance and ethics. Available at: https://www.hcpc-uk.org/standards/standards-of-conduct-performance-and-ethics/ [Accessed 2024-11-21].

CHAPTER 4

Opportunities for Global Collaboration in Radiation Oncology: The Radiation Planning Assistant as a Case Study

Laurence Court and William Shaw

4.1 CHAPTER OBJECTIVES

- To explore the mechanisms and benefits of global collaboration in radiation oncology

- To use the Radiation Planning Assistant as a case study

- To examine collaborations from the following perspectives

  - Achievement of diverse goals

  - Various roles in collaborative projects

  - Team sizes

  - Timeframes

  - Organizational types

DOI: 10.1201/9781003527749-4

- Intersection of global collaborations with career development
- To consider actionable insights
- To provide recommendations for fostering impactful partnerships

4.2 THE RADIATION PLANNING ASSISTANT: BACKGROUND

It is estimated that, by 2040, 70% of annual cancer cases are projected to occur in low- and middle-income countries (LMICs), yet fewer than 50% of patients in these regions have access to radiotherapy [1]. Alarmingly, approximately 80% of the world's cancer patients rely on just 5% of global radiotherapy resources [2]. According to the Lancet Oncology Commission, addressing this disparity could save nearly one million lives annually [1]. However, achieving this goal would require an estimated 50,000 additional radiation oncologists and medical physicists. Alongside workforce recruitment and training, enhancing workflow efficiency is critical to enabling clinical teams to treat more patients while managing costs and resource limitations. Automation, including artificial intelligence, presents a promising opportunity to narrow the gap in radiotherapy access and quality. Improved efficiency not only enhances care but also increases the return on investment in radiotherapy infrastructure [1, 3].

With this context, the Radiation Planning Assistant (RPA) project was initiated in 2015 and received funding in 2016 [4]. Its goal is to leverage automated contouring (identifying treatment targets and normal tissues on CT scans) and treatment planning (designing the position, intensity, and shape of radiation beams) to assist oncologists in LMICs. This support enables oncologists to expand their capacity, treating more patients safely and efficiently while improving access to care. The initiative focuses on developing a comprehensive suite of automated planning tools tailored for various tumour types and treatment indications. To ensure their suitability for LMIC settings, these tools have been co-developed in collaboration with clinical teams from South Africa, the Philippines, Tanzania, the United Kingdom, and the United States [5]. These collaborations have involved teams of clinical staff (radiation oncologists, physicists, treatment planners), as well as programmers, research assistants, trainees, and others. This project has been funded by institutional sources (MD Anderson Cancer Center), as well as with national and state grants [US National Cancer Institute (NCI), Cancer Prevention and Research Institute of Texas

CPRIT)], vendors (Varian), and foundations (Wellcome Trust). It has provided teams across the world (high- and low-income countries) the opportunity to grow through collaboration, and to contribute on a global scale in a way that would not normally be possible. In this chapter, we use the RPA as a case study to describe various aspects of global collaborations.

4.3 THE RADIATION PLANNING ASSISTANT: TIMELINE

Below is a summary of the RPA project timeline as it grew from an idea to a small project, eventually becoming a medium-sized project. The next steps will be to scale the RPA to more countries, adding more capabilities.

2014: Visit to South Africa. Three members of the (future) RPA team visited several hospitals in South Africa to propose and discuss the RPA project, and to understand whether it is really a good idea or simply a cute physics project. Decision made to submit a proposal to the US National Cancer Institute (NCI).

2015: Visit to the Philippines. Another site visit to further discuss possibilities.

2015: NCI proposal submitted.

2016: Notice of Award received, project formally started with two graduate students and a programmer.

2021: Quality Management Plan (QMP) v1 go-live. This was part of our progression to a professional team, with appropriate quality and risk management, and software development processes.

2022: MD Anderson (MDA) Global Oncology Program launched. This brought the RPA project much more in alignment with the MDA's global strategy.

2023: FDA 510(k) clearance for the RPA. Approval by the US Food and Drug Administration (FDA) demonstrating a reasonable assurance for safety and effectiveness.

2023: MDA's leadership announces the goal of making the RPA available for free to clinics that would not otherwise have access to similar tools.

2023: QMP v2. Updates to our original QMP to better accommodate responses to customers and other items.

2024: Largest collaborative work published, showing clinical accept-
ability scoring from 31 radiation oncologists at 16 institutions in six
countries [5].

2024: Legal approval for South Africa (terms of use, etc.) and go-live.

The many global collaborations that have resulted from this work have led
to around 80 scientific papers and other publications and involved more
than 15 trainees.

4.3.1 Research

Research in radiation oncology is vital for advancing cancer treatment
and for improving access to radiation therapy across the world. The development and validation of the RPA required extensive collaboration across
institutions. This started with extensive discussions on clinical workflows,
treatment approaches, and potential risks. Later, research collaborations
ensured that the tool's algorithms were tested in a variety of clinical sce-
narios, from simple treatment plans to complex cases. Multi-institutional
studies contributed to the validation of RPA-generated plans against
those created by experienced dosimetrists. These collaborations not only
improved the RPA's functionality but also created opportunities for publications and grant funding, benefiting all parties involved.

4.3.2 Education and Training

One of the primary goals of global collaboration is the advancement of
education and training in radiation oncology. In fact, the majority of
global collaborations seem to involve training, rather than research. In
all projects, there may be an explicit education and training goal, such as
developing a training course; alternatively, training may happen as part of
a research project, where the active involvement of trainees in the project
development and execution is part of their training. Thus, most projects
have an educational aspect. The project leadership should carefully design
the team so that trainees on all sides of the collaboration benefit.

The RPA project has involved many trainees, mostly graduate students
at MDA. They have developed prototypes of various autocontouring and
autoplanning tools, typically working with radiation oncologists in other
institutions. This level of collaboration has provided an introduction to
variations in clinical practice across the world and the differing needs of
different clinics, especially those in LMICs. Some trainees were also able

to visit South Africa, further enhancing their understanding of radiation therapy in other countries. When we started this project, education/training was not an explicit goal of the project, but most projects will involve trainees, and this should be considered and planned from the project initiation. Involvement of more trainees in our collaborating centres would also have provided additional educational benefits.

Collaborative efforts, such as partnerships between academic institutions and professional organizations like the American Association of Physicists in Medicine (AAPM), or international agencies like the International Atomic Energy Agency (IAEA), can also enhance the educational and training opportunities, including fellowships, which will help build a future workforce with an understanding of global oncology.

4.3.3 Clinical Service

Another focus of global collaborations can be on clinical service. For example, clinical teams who are experienced in a particular treatment approach (e.g., brachytherapy) may visit a hospital to share these experiences. This is very common and can be extremely valuable to the recipient team. Clinical service collaborations can take many forms, including individual visits, short courses, and weekly seminars focusing on clinical or technical aspects of radiation oncology. An excellent example of this is Project ECHO (Extension for Community Healthcare Outcomes), a tele-mentoring programme that brings people together for knowledge exchange [6].

The RPA project team has worked with local teams to optimize the RPA workflows and artificial intelligence (AI) models to try to provide tools that work in different clinical environments/workflows and with different patient populations. This involves working with the clinical teams to share data and experiences, as well as testing all aspects of the tool. Collaborative efforts to implement the RPA in LMICs further require understanding local needs, especially of the multidisciplinary teams (oncologists, physicists, treatment planners) that are involved in RPA deployment.

4.4 COLLABORATION WITH DIFFERENT PERSONNEL POSITIONS

4.4.1 Research Staff

Research staff play a pivotal role in collaborative projects like the RPA. They contribute to algorithm development, validation studies, and data analysis. In the case of the RPA, international collaborations allowed research teams to access anonymized treatment planning data from diverse patient populations, enriching the tool's development and global applicability. Our programmers have visited other hospitals to gain an improved understanding of their needs (motivation) and have worked closely with physicists and radiation oncologists. In addition to improving the output of the project, these collaborations have also enriched our research teams with motivation, novel new projects, and overall excitement and commitment to the projects that would probably not have happened without the close collaborations.

4.4.2   Clinical Staff

Clinical staff are integral to many projects, especially those like the RPA. In the early stages, their involvement is essential when trying to understand local needs, patient populations, and clinical approaches. Later, their feedback ensures that the tool is user-friendly and meets clinical needs. Clinicians participating in RPA-related collaborations often act as trainers in a two-way process – variations in experience, patient populations, and available equipment mean that we all have something to learn from each other.

4.4.3   Trainees and Small Teams

Trainees, including residents and fellows, benefit significantly from collaborative projects. Exposure to tools like the RPA enhances their understanding of clinical processes and treatment planning, and introduces them to global oncology challenges. In turn, trainees contribute fresh perspectives and innovative solutions to collaborative efforts.

4.5   COLLABORATION THROUGH DIFFERENT TEAM SIZES

4.5.1   Individuals

Individual contributors play a foundational role in global collaborations. For instance, a physicist might volunteer to visit a clinic in a low-income country to share their expertise. They may also support a larger project, like the RPA, by supporting implementation in a specific clinic, perhaps one where they have already developed a relationship with the physics and oncology teams. Such contributions have a profound impact on the success of larger initiatives.

4.5.2   Mentoring and Teaching

Mentoring and teaching are essential for the sustainability of global collaborations. Senior clinicians and physicists often mentor local staff, building their capacity to independently use and adapt the tool. This mentorship model ensures long-term success and fosters cross-cultural professional relationships. (Also, see Chapter 8 on Mentoring in the Global Context.)

4.5.3 Consulting

Consulting services are another avenue for collaboration. Experts in radiation oncology may be consulted to guide the integration of the RPA into existing clinical workflows. These collaborations often involve addressing challenges such as regulatory compliance, technical infrastructure, and staff training.

4.5.4 Teams and Multi-Institutional Collaboration

Larger teams and multi-institutional collaborations are critical for projects of the RPA's scale. These teams bring together diverse expertise, including software developers, radiation oncologists, and medical physicists. Multi-institutional collaborations, such as clinical trials comparing RPA-generated plans to conventional ones, ensure that the tool meets international standards and is widely accepted.

4.6 COLLABORATION THROUGH DIFFERENT TIMEFRAMES

4.6.1 Short-Term Projects

Short-term collaborations, such as "voluntourism" initiatives, provide immediate support for clinics. Volunteers might travel to a clinic to train staff or troubleshoot technical issues. While impactful, these collaborations require careful planning to ensure sustainability. It is important that these projects are real projects, developed together with the local clinical team, and not just an excuse to visit somewhere new.

4.6.2 Medium-Term Projects

Many larger projects, which are initially developed as medium-term projects (projects that start because of success in a grant submission to a national institution such as the NIH), are good examples of these, as they are typically three to five years in length. The RPA is a good example of a project that started as a medium-term project. This is the time where relationships are built. Although Zoom meetings are useful in maintaining relationships, we have found that actual in-person visits are essential to keeping projects moving forward, and also offer the best opportunities to understand local situations and challenges.

4.6.3 Long-Term Projects

Long-term collaborations almost always start as medium-term projects that are sufficiently successful for them to continue and, in most cases, expand to additional collaborations, scaling the project impact. The RPA project started in 2016, and has now evolved into a long-term project. This transition requires a new focus on establishing sustainable systems, including personnel and funding models. Specifically, this involves additional collaborations with new clinics, expanding to new countries, as well as ongoing training and continuous software updates. Scaling may also involve partnerships with international agencies like the World Health Organization (WHO) or the IAEA.

4.7 COLLABORATION THROUGH DIFFERENT TYPES OF ORGANIZATIONS

4.7.1 Academic Institutions

Academic institutions are central to the development and validation of the RPA. We have developed many relationships through these projects. All institutions have their own bureaucracy and ways of doing things, and patience is definitely needed when processing contracts, protocols, and data transfer agreements. However, if you persevere, this is almost always worth the effort, as these collaborations can be extremely productive and satisfying.

4.7.2 Industry Partnerships

Industry partnerships can take many levels, from relatively low-level support (basic technical support, letters of support for grant applications), through in-kind loans (e.g., research treatment planning systems, other equipment), to active collaboration through academic industry partnerships (AIPs), Small Business Innovation Research (SBIR) projects, and others. Depending on the project, and the need for widespread implementation and uptake, industry support may actually be essential. (Also, see Chapter 5 on Global Collaborations with Industry.)

The RPA project has had support from Varian Medical Systems for most of its development lifecycle, starting with a letter of support during the initial NCI grant submission, to a much larger research grant to expand the RPA portfolio, and even to a letter of support when we submitted the RPA to the FDA for 510(k) approval. For this particular project, this level of support has been essential; without it, the project would not have reached the level of success that it has.

4.7.3 Collaboration through Professional and Other Organizations

Professional organizations, such as the AAPM, International Cancer Expert Corps (ICEC), and RAD-AID, play a crucial role in promoting global collaboration. They provide platforms for sharing knowledge, coordinating efforts, and securing funding. In some cases, they can even provide funding (e.g., fellowships) to support projects in their early stages. The RPA project has had minimal involvement with these organizations, but we suggest involvement would have been helpful, especially for trainees who are developing their global health careers. A sample list of relevant organizations can be found in Chapter 17 on Global Collaborating Organizations.

4.8 FUNDING OF INTERNATIONAL COLLABORATIONS

International collaborations are often funded with a complex web of funding sources, likely a combination of NIH (or similar), foundations, industry, and other sources. The RPA project was initiated with funding from the NIH. That initial grant was made possible by our collaboration with Varian Medical Systems, which later added additional funding to the project. We later leveraged our success to obtain funding from the Wellcome Trust and the Cancer Prevention Research Institute of Texas (CPRIT).

It is important to maintain equity in funding, so that the funding is not just for the collaborator in the high-income country. We have learned that this is not as simple as it may sound and requires careful discussion between the collaborators.

Especially for those living in the United States, a good starting point when looking for funding for global health projects is the NCI Center for Global Health: cancer.gov/about-nci/organization/cgh/funding. Other sources of funding can be found on the webpages of the various professional organizations summarized in Chapter 17.

4.9 GLOBAL COLLABORATIONS AND CAREER DEVELOPMENT

New faculty who are considering a career in global health are generally led by their desire to improve healthcare across the world. They should, however, also consider their own career development. Institutional leaders should also consider this as they mentor new staff. Individual expectations need to be met, but so do the institutions' expectations, especially those regarding career progression and promotion.

4.9.1 Individual Expectations

Global collaborations provide opportunities for career development by enabling individuals to gain expertise in specific areas, such as automated treatment planning. Professionals involved in the RPA project often become recognized experts, enhancing their national and international reputations. Also, these projects can be a lot of fun – it is always best to do a project that you enjoy!

4.9.2 Institutional Expectations

Institutions benefit from their staff's participation in global collaborations. Success in initiatives like the RPA contributes to an institution's reputation for excellence in clinical service, research, and training. Publications, funding, and recognition in professional circles further enhance institutional prestige. For most medical physicists in academic centres, their promotion prospects centre around excellence in clinical service, research, and teaching. If their institution does not explicitly acknowledge contributions to global health, they may need to show their successes in different ways, e.g., by submitting papers on their collaborative projects in/with LMICs.

Even if the collaboration is not a research project, there are other types of papers that are useful to the community (as well as to the individual for their promotion). Examples include needs assessment and comparison of different treatment approaches in different environments or countries. For example, as part of the RPA project, several papers have been accepted looking at the hurdles in the use of the RPA (based on surveys of potential users) and on local evaluation of RPA tools. Collaborative projects can also lead to invited conference presentations, e.g., members of the RPA team have been invited to present at the annual meeting of the South African Association of Physicists in Medicine and Biology – these are both fun for the individual and great support for academic promotion. Individuals need to consider these to plan for their long-term success in global collaborations.

4.9.3 Networking Opportunities

Participating in global collaborations offers valuable networking opportunities. Professionals involved in the RPA project often build relationships with colleagues from international agencies, paving the way for future partnerships and career advancement.

4.10 SUMMARY AND RECOMMENDATIONS

4.10.1 Summary

By examining the Radiation Planning Assistant as a case study, this chapter has highlighted the potential of global collaboration in radiation oncology. Through coordinated efforts, diverse expertise, and a shared commitment to improving care, we can address global disparities and advance the field.

4.10.2 Recommendations

Based on the last eight years of RPA projects, we have the following recommendations for global collaborations. Some of these we knew from the start. Most of these were learned the hard way.

1. **Foster Multi-Institutional Partnerships**: Encourage collaborations between academic institutions, industry, and international agencies to enhance the development and implementation of tools like the RPA. Initiating projects is relatively straightforward, but relationships require continual care and attention. We attribute one of the reasons for the success of the collaborations established through the RPA project to consistent and frequent site visits with each other (at least one site visit per year).

2. **Invest in Training and Capacity Building**: Prioritize training programmes that equip local staff with the skills needed to use and adapt new technologies.

3. **Ensure Sustainability**: Design projects with long-term sustainability in mind, including ongoing support and software updates, as well as sustainable funding. Although you don't know how successful the project will be when you start, be ready to pivot towards sustainability when you find the project is going well! Site visits to discuss the project with peers before starting a project will also help ensure you embark on a useful project.

4. **Leverage Professional Organizations**: Utilize platforms provided by organizations like the AAPM and RAD-AID to coordinate efforts and share best practices. This may be especially useful when initially establishing relationships, and then again if your project starts to scale and you need additional support.

5. **Align with Global Health Goals**: Collaborate with international agencies to ensure that initiatives like the RPA contribute to broader public health objectives, such as equitable access to cancer care. It is also necessary to align with your institutional goals, e.g., the RPA project

has aligned itself with the Global Oncology focus of the MD Anderson Cancer Center, thus ensuring institutional support as we move forward.

6. **Measure Impact**: Regularly evaluate the impact of collaborative efforts on patient outcomes, clinical workflows, and professional development to guide future initiatives. We are very used to measuring effectiveness (e.g., quantitative comparison of automatic and manual contours), but in order to impact human health, other outcomes, specifically service and implementation outcomes [7] (time saved, adoption, etc.), must also be measured.

REFERENCES

1. Atun, R., *et al.*, Expanding global access to radiotherapy. *The Lancet Oncology*, 2015. **16**(10): p. 1153–1186.
2. Farmer, P., et al., Expansion of cancer care and control in countries of low and middle income: a call to action. *The Lancet*, 2010. **376**(9747): p. 1186–1193.
3. Ngwa, W., et al., Cancer in sub-Saharan Africa: a Lancet Oncology Commission. *The Lancet Oncology*, 2022. **23**(6): p. e251-e312.
4. Court, L.E., The Radiation Planning Assistant: addressing the global gap in radiotherapy services. *The Lancet Oncology*, 2024. **25**(3): p. 277-278.
5. Court, L.E., *et al.*, Artificial Intelligence-Based Radiotherapy Contouring and Planning to Improve Global Access to Cancer Care. *JCO Global Oncology*, 2024. **10**: p. e2300376.
6. Varon, M.L., *et al.*, Project ECHO cancer initiative: a tool to improve care and increase capacity along the continuum of cancer care. *Journal of Cancer Education*, 2021. **36**(1): p. 25–38.
7. Proctor, E., *et al.*, Outcomes for implementation research: conceptual distinctions, measurement challenges, and research agenda. *Administration and Policy in Mental Health and Mental Health Services Research*, 2011. **38**(2): p. 65–76.

CHAPTER 5

Global Collaborations with Industry

Jennifer Dent, Cathyryne Manner, and Katy Graef

5.1 CHAPTER OBJECTIVES

- To describe the benefits of industry collaborations

- To describe types of industry collaborations

- To describe methods of fostering effective industry/cross-sector collaborations

- To provide recommendations on Global Medical Physics collaborations with industry

5.2 INTRODUCTION

Industry collaborations – commonly referred to as public–private partnerships – unite the diverse expertise, perspectives, resources, and programme management approaches of for-profit companies, government organizations, academic institutions, and non-profit organizations to achieve shared objectives. Public–private partnerships have the potential to accomplish what no individual organization could achieve alone. Industry partnerships also have the benefit of expanding resources, including financial investments, and distributing programme risks.

In global health, industry collaborations that bring together low- and middle-income country (LMIC) stakeholders and international partners

DOI: 10.1201/9781003527749-5

are vital for catalyzing basic and clinical research, building scientific and healthcare professional capacity, strengthening infrastructure, and delivering access to quality healthcare services.

LMIC partners must be at the forefront of all global health initiatives and partnerships. These partners provide essential insights and first-hand knowledge to ensure alignment with local priorities, and acceptance, uptake, and sustainability of collaboration outcomes. Private sector collaborators – including medical device, diagnostic, technology, biotechnology, and pharmaceutical companies – bring equipment, systems, software, and experience incorporating products into healthcare systems. Government agencies and academic partners bring the knowledge and build the skills to implement and operate systems that advance research and healthcare. Together, these partners provide the critical resources needed to deliver healthcare to patients.

This chapter describes methods, best practices, and lessons learned for developing and managing global collaborations with industry, which are applicable across technological and therapeutic areas. In particular, we highlight global oncology and Global Medical Physics collaborations with industry as model programmes that deliver substantial value and impact.

5.3 ADDRESSING AFRICA'S CANCER CRISIS THROUGH GLOBAL MEDICAL PHYSICS COLLABORATIONS WITH INDUSTRY

Cancer is an escalating health problem in Africa that will require industry partnership to curb the current trend. In 2022, more Africans died from cancer than from AIDS-related illnesses, and Africa's cancer mortality-to-incidence ratio (0.64) was more than double the ratio (0.25) in the United States [1, 2]. The annual number of new cancer cases in Africa is projected to increase by nearly 80% by 2040 [3].

Limited access to quality health services across the continuum of care – prevention, screening, detection, diagnosis, and treatment – is a key driver of Africa's cancer crisis. Many cancers are diagnosed at late stages, contributing to poor patient outcomes, for reasons including barriers to healthcare services and inadequate diagnostic capacity [4]. In addition to late presentation of disease, a shortage of skilled personnel, especially in advanced specialty areas such as radiotherapy, limits the critical services needed to deliver treatment to cancer patients. Radiotherapy patient services require advanced technologies and specialized skills to operate and maintain these complex systems. The costs of operating these systems and facilities are substantial, which contribute to the challenges of delivering radiotherapy services [5].

Global Medical Physics companies are for-profit enterprises engaged in research and development (R&D), manufacturing, sales, and distribution of medical physics products and services in international markets. These companies play important roles in combatting Africa's cancer crisis in collaboration with African and other international partners. Such companies leverage their material and intellectual resources to advance:

- **R&D:** Clinical trials and other studies to validate medical physics technologies in African patients – technologies that previously may have been tested only in high-income countries with different ethnic makeups.

- **Human capacity development:** Training programmes to (a) empower African healthcare providers to utilize medical physics equipment to care for cancer patients, and (b) equip African scientists with the skills and capabilities to conduct high-quality Global Medical Physics research.

- **Infrastructure development and product access:** Expansion of access to medical physics products in African countries and healthcare facilities.

Public–private partnerships enable Global Medical Physics companies to reach more patients globally – including in underserved communities – and deliver substantial health impacts. These partnerships include the International Atomic Energy Agency (IAEA)'s Rays of Hope initiative, which helps Member States establish and expand radiotherapy and medical imaging capacities through training, equipment, and facilities construction. According to an analysis by the Lancet Oncology Commission on Medical Imaging and Nuclear Medicine, comprehensive scale-up of imaging, radiotherapy, and other treatment modalities (chemotherapy, surgery, and targeted therapy) between 2020 and 2030 in Africa would avert 2.5 million cancer deaths and save 61.3 million life-years [6]. Industry collaborations also address Corporate Social Responsibility (CSR) and Environmental, Social, and Governance (ESG) objectives and support commercial opportunities within emerging markets of strategic importance.

5.4 FOSTERING GLOBAL INDUSTRY COLLABORATIONS

5.4.1 Effective Industry Partnership Models

Customized, proactive approaches to establishing and managing three types of LMIC-driven industry collaborations are described in Table 5.1. These partnership development and alliance management approaches have been implemented, evaluated, and adapted over two decades by BIO Ventures for Global Health (BVGH) to optimize outcomes, partner experiences, and limit risks associated with public–private partnerships [7–12].

5.4.2 Monitoring, Evaluation, and Reporting

Monitoring, evaluating, and reporting collaboration outcomes and impacts to partners and targeted external audiences (such as mainstream media, the public, United Nations agencies, and United States Congress) are critical for fostering transparency and trust; expanding positive visibility and recognition; and attracting new partners and funders. Sample metrics for each type of collaboration are summarized in Table 5.2.

TABLE 5.1   BVGH Partnering and Alliance Management Approaches

Type of Collaboration	Methods
R&D	• **Assess:** Analyze R&D goals and collaboration interests of LMIC partners, including scientific/technology focus; research stage (e.g., clinical validation); and specific expertise or assets needed. • **Search and match**: Identify international entities with complementary interests and resources. • **Connect:** Introduce LMIC stakeholders to international entities. Coordinate non-confidential discussions to confirm mutual interest in collaborating. • **Partner:** Facilitate relationship development. Align on collaboration milestones, timelines, deliverables, budgets, key performance indicators (KPIs), and responsibilities. Support negotiation and execution of legal agreements. • **Manage:** Provide end-to-end alliance management support for collaborations. Coordinate routine meetings, and check in remotely between meetings, to track progress and ensure communication is maintained, expectations are aligned, milestones and obligations are met, and challenges are resolved. Update milestones and engage new partners as needed. • **Fund:** Help partners identify external funding opportunities through BVGH FundFinder and develop competitive proposals by, for example, reviewing and advising on draft proposals and providing letters of support.

(Continued)

TABLE 5.1 *(Continued)*

Human capacity development	• **Assess:** Define training needs with LMIC partners, including preferred languages.
	• **Plan:** Align on training programme formats with LMIC leaders and trainees, based on considerations including the need for hands-on instruction (e.g., use of imaging or radiotherapy equipment). Effective training formats include:
	  • Seminar series: Digital (lectures and discussions over several weeks) and in-person (3–4 days of presentations and discussions).
	  • Virtual mentorship platforms (VMPs): Online venues for LMIC professionals and international experts to discuss topics of mutual interest; share lessons learned and best practices; and address challenges.
	  • Fellowships: Placements of international experts at LMIC facilities and LMIC professionals at international organizations.
	• **Implement:**
	  • All programmes (as applicable): Engage international trainers and mentors; support their preparations (e.g., materials development). Create agendas/training plans. Set up and manage virtual platforms (e.g., Zoom) and onsite venues. Coordinate travel and logistics. Conduct pre- and post-training assessments.
	  • Seminar series: Host and moderate sessions. Publish and promote training materials through LMIC and international channels.
	  • VMPs: Schedule and facilitate regular online exchanges between LMIC professionals and mentors. Ensure active engagement by all, including regular postings on the platform.
	  • Fellowships: Match LMIC professionals and mentors. Determine fellowship locations (LMIC and/or mentor facilities). Facilitate relationship development. Align on milestones, timelines, deliverables, budgets, KPIs, and responsibilities. Provide end-to-end alliance management support as described above for R&D collaborations.

Infrastructure development and product access	• **Forecast demand:** In collaboration with LMIC partners, forecast numbers of patients eligible for care using the target products (including imaging systems, radiotherapy machines, and radioisotopes). Determine if any other products, services, or infrastructure are required to safely provide appropriate care. Leveraging these data, forecast quarterly and annual demand for the target products and engage other partners (including entities such as IAEA's Rays of Hope initiative) as needed to address other product, service, or infrastructure gaps.

(Continued)

TABLE 5.1 (*Continued*)

- **Develop access and payer models:** Engage LMIC governments; funding agencies, and national organizations investing in healthcare; and healthcare facilities to co-develop and pilot programmes that drive and scale access to the target products. Use regional and patient-level socioeconomic data to develop a patient poverty index and a tiered pricing model to stratify patients based on their ability to afford the target products and any other needed products or services.
- **Coordinate procurement and delivery:** Coordinate and streamline direct purchase agreements with product manufacturers. Eliminate unnecessary intermediaries and price mark-ups. Facilitate expedited product registration (or regulatory waivers until registration is complete) and importation. Secure supply chains. Ensure compliance with regulatory and customs requirements. Maintain oversight and tracking of products from Port to Patient. (Healthcare facilities are responsible for medical monitoring.)

TABLE 5.2 Collaboration Metrics

Type of Collaboration	Sample Metrics
R&D	- Collaborations established.
	- LMIC scientists and international industry, government, academic, and non-profit partners engaged.
	- Key milestones achieved.
	- New joint R&D activities established as a result of collaborations.
	- Peer-reviewed publications produced.
	- Grant funding secured by LMIC scientists.
	- International recognition received by LMIC scientists (e.g., speaking opportunities at global meetings; media coverage).
	- Promotions or other career accolades for LMIC scientists received.
Human capacity development	- Training programmes completed.
	- LMIC professionals trained.
	- Skills developed or skill gaps addressed.
	- Improvements in trainees' knowledge and confidence in training topics.
	- Application of learnings – by trainees, and colleagues with whom they share their learnings – to advance R&D and improve patient care and outcomes.
Infrastructure development and product access	- Purchase agreements executed.
	- Quantities of target products purchased and delivered to LMIC healthcare facilities.
	- Patients cared for with the target products.
	- Improvements in patient outcomes attributable to target products.

5.5 GLOBAL INDUSTRY COLLABORATION CASE STUDIES

BVGH has forged and managed public–private partnerships for 20 years to solve global health issues. Selected case studies are presented below.

5.5.1 HypoAfrica [5]

Hypofractionated radiotherapy (HFRT) offers promise as an economical solution to treatment access barriers in LMICs [13]. However, most studies highlighting HFRT's benefits for cancer treatment have been conducted in Western patients. Through the BVGH-led African Access Initiative (AAI) and African Consortium for Cancer Clinical Trials (AC³T), BVGH organized a team of African principal investigators and expert advisors from Australia, Europe, and the United States to assess the feasibility of implementing HFRT for prostate cancer in sub-Saharan Africa. The HypoAfrica Phase II multi-centre study launched in 2022 and is ongoing as of October 2024 with sites participating from four African countries: Nigeria, South Africa, Tanzania, and Uganda. The primary endpoints of the study are toxicity at the end of treatment and at 3–24 months post-treatment. Secondary endpoints are prostate-specific antigen failure-free survival at 5 years, relapse-free survival at 5 years, overall survival at 5 years, and HFRT cost-effectiveness. The collaborators have gleaned valuable insights into barriers to HFRT implementation – in the HypoAfrica trial, and Africa more broadly. These barriers are addressed through the consortium's weekly meetings – facilitated and managed by BVGH – which include troubleshooting equipment and software technical issues, developing or sharing standard operating procedures (SOPs), addressing safety concerns, conducting educational lectures, and sharing members' experiences. The HypoAfrica team has presented study data at multiple international conferences, published in peer-reviewed journals, and submitted grant applications to build on the strength and experience of this public–private medical physicist partnership. Takeda Pharmaceuticals provided the seed funding to launch this study and consortium, which has proven to be sustainable beyond the initial funds.

5.5.2 Diagnostic Imaging Digital Training Programme

Nano-X Imaging Ltd (Nanox) sponsored AAI with the aim of expanding imaging knowledge and capacity in Africa. BVGH collaborated with Nigerian AAI partners to gain an understanding of the current imaging capacity and training priorities. With this information in hand, BVGH developed and implemented a two-part, 12-session digital webinar series that trained hundreds of LMIC professionals – primarily African – on ultrasound, X-ray, computed tomography (CT), CT-guided interventional procedures, positron emission tomography/CT imaging, breast magnetic resonance imaging, and tomosynthesis. Lectures were developed and delivered virtually by experts from Nanox, Emory University School of Medicine, Memorial Sloan Kettering Cancer Center, Penn Medicine, RAD-AID Kenya, RAD-AID Nigeria, and USARAD. BVGH also coordinated a customized mentorship for webinar participants at a Nigerian medical centre. The Nigerian professionals and their mentor – a radiologist at a renowned United States medical centre – co-developed and are applying for grant funding for a programme to train Nigerian radiologists in the diagnosis of deep vein thrombosis and peripheral artery disease.

5.5.3 Intensity-Modulated Radiation Therapy (IMRT) Digital Training Programmes

In collaboration with Rayos Contra Cancer (RCC), a non-profit organization established and led by academic medical physicists and radiation oncologists, BVGH coordinated an AAI IMRT webinar series for Anglophone and Francophone radiation oncologists, medical physicists, and radiotherapy technicians in LMICs. RCC has a longstanding partnership with the Elekta Foundation, which provides funding and support for its programmes, including digital training.

5.5.4 Brachytherapy Infrastructure and Capacity Strengthening

At the request of the Nigeria Sovereign Investment Authority-Lagos University Teaching Hospital Cancer Center (NLCC), BVGH supported the centre's commissioning and launching of the site's 3D high dose-rate (HDR) brachytherapy, initially for the treatment of cervical cancer patients. BVGH connected the NLCC radiotherapy team with medical physics experts from Calvary Mater Newcastle Public Hospital, New South Wales, Australia, and Kaiser Permanente, USA, to guide NLCC's brachytherapy preparations, including advising on applicator commissioning and pre-treatment quality assurance calculations and procedures using Gafchromic film. Due to the limited availability of cost-effective Gafchromic film in Africa, BVGH purchased the film in the USA and shipped it to Nigeria. Once preparations were complete, BVGH arranged for a medical physicist from Varian Medical Systems and a radiation oncologist from Ahmad Bin Zayed Al Nahyan Center for Cancer

Treatment in Morocco to travel to Lagos, Nigeria, to initiate clinical treatment with the 3D HDR brachytherapy system. During their time in Lagos at NLCC, the two experts commissioned the brachytherapy equipment, practised the brachytherapy workflow with the NLCC staff, and administered brachytherapy to NLCC patients while training the team. Following the hands-on training, BVGH organized a post-commissioning virtual review between an expert from the University of California San Diego and NLCC to refine the centre's methods to calculate the biologically effective dose of radiotherapy, use of dose shaper and dwell control window, creation of customized reports, scheduling of patient treatments, and the use of needle applications. Collaborators involved in this project enabled NLCC to operationalize their significant infrastructure investment and project, while positioning the healthcare team to provide treatment to their patients.

5.6 SUMMARY AND RECOMMENDATIONS

5.6.1 Summary

Industry collaborations, or public–private partnerships, that merge and align the complementary expertise and resources of companies, governments, academia, and non-profit organizations are critical for accomplishing common goals that no single sector can accomplish independently. In global health – including Global Medical Physics – such collaborations, when driven by LMIC priorities, have the power to:

- Catalyze critical R&D, including clinical trials.

- Build human capacity in research and clinical care.

- Strengthen infrastructure and expand access to lifesaving products.

Methodology and best practices for developing and managing industry collaborations are applicable across technological and therapeutic areas. However, Global Medical Physics collaborations with industry in the field of global oncology can deliver substantial value and impact.

5.6.2 Recommendations

Global Medical Physics stakeholders interested in participating in industry collaborations should adhere to the following key principles and drivers of collaboration success:

- Focus on addressing the self-defined needs and priorities of LMIC partners.

- Engagement and buy-in at the highest levels of each partner organization.

- Mutual respect for organizational and cultural differences, such as communication styles, healthcare-seeking behaviours, and levels of trust in conventional healthcare systems.

- Alignment of all partners on concrete milestones, timelines, roles, and responsibilities.

- Robust monitoring, evaluation, and reporting frameworks.

  - Internal reporting fosters transparency, trust, and prompt identification and resolution of issues.

  - External reporting increases positive visibility and helps attract new partners and funders.

Global Medical Physics professionals who are new to industry collaborations can benefit from guidance and partnership with experienced organizations.

REFERENCES

1. Ferlay J, Ervik M, Lam F, Laversanne M, Colombet M, Mery L, Piñeros M, Znaor A, Soerjomataram I, Bray F (2024). Global Cancer Observatory: Cancer Today (version 1.1). Lyon, France: International Agency for Research on Cancer. Available from: https://gco.iarc.who.int/today, accessed 15 October 2024.
2. World Health Organization Regional Office for Africa. Health Topics: HIV/AIDS. https://www.afro.who.int/health-topics/hivaids
3. Ferlay J, Laversanne M, Ervik M, Lam F, Colombet M, Mery L, Piñeros M, Znaor A, Soerjomataram I, Bray F (2024). Global Cancer Observatory: Cancer Tomorrow (version 1.1). Lyon, France: International Agency for Research on Cancer. Available from: https://gco.iarc.who.int/tomorrow [Accessed on 2024-11-14].
4. Ngwa W, Addai BW, Adewole I, Ainsworth V, Alaro J, Alatise OI, Ali Z, Anderson BO, Anorlu R, Avery S, Barango P, Bih N, Booth CM, Brawley OW, Dangou JM, Denny L, Dent J, Elmore SNC, Elzawawy A, Gashumba D, Geel J, Graef K, Gupta S, Gueye SM, Hammad N, Hessissen L, Ilbawi AM, Kambugu J, Kozlakidis Z, Manga S, Maree L, Mohammed SI, Msadabwe S, Mutebi M, Nakaganda A, Ndlovu N, Ndoh K, Ndumbalo J, Ngoma M, Ngoma T, Ntizimira C, Rebbeck TR, Renner L, Romanoff A, Rubagumya F,

Sayed S, Sud S, Simonds H, Sullivan R, Swanson W, Vanderpuye V, Wiafe B, Kerr D. Cancer in Sub-Saharan Africa: A Lancet Oncology Commission. *Lancet Oncol.* 2022 Jun;23(6):e251–e312.

5. Olatunji E, Swanson W, Patel S, Adeneye SO, Aina-Tofolari F, Avery S, Kisukari JD, Graef K, Huq S, Jeraj R, Joseph AO, Lehmann J, Li H, Mallum A, Mkhize T, Ngoma TA, Studen A, Wijesooriya K, Incrocci L, Ngwa W. Challenges and Opportunities for Implementing Hypofractionated Radiotherapy in Africa: Lessons from the HypoAfrica Clinical Trial. *Ecancermedicalscience.* 2023 Feb 16;17:1508.

6. Hricak H, Abdel-Wahab M, Atun R, Lette MM, Paez D, Brink JA, Donoso-Bach L, Frija G, Hierath M, Holmberg O, Khong PL, Lewis JS, McGinty G, Oyen WJG, Shulman LN, Ward ZJ, Scott AM. Medical Imaging and Nuclear Medicine: A Lancet Oncology Commission. *Lancet Oncol.* 2021 Apr;22(4):e136–e172.

7. Seymour DJL, Graef KM, Iliyasu Y, Diomande MIJM, Jaquet S, Kelly M, Soles R, Milner DA. Pathology Training for Cancer Diagnosis in Africa. *Am J Clin Pathol.* 2022 Feb 3;157(2):279–285.

8. Graef KM, Okoye I, Ohene Oti NO, Dent J, Odedina FT. Operational Strategies for Clinical Trials in Africa. *JCO Glob Oncol.* 2020 Jun;6:973–982.

9. Manner CK, Graef KM, Dent J. WIPO Re:Search: Catalyzing Public-Private Partnerships to Accelerate Tropical Disease Drug Discovery and Development. *Trop Med Infect Dis.* 2019 Mar 26;4(1):53.

10. Estes C. Building a Cancer Center around Patients in Nigeria. *Bio News*, July 19, 2022. Available from: https://bio.news/health/building-a-cancer-center-around-patients-in-nigeria/ [Accessed on 2024-11-14].

11. Estes C. "BVGH AC³T Is Changing Lives, One Clinical Trial at a Time. *Bio News*, April 21, 2022. Available from: https://bio.news/health/bvgh-ac%C2%B3t-is-changing-lives-one-clinical-trial-at-a-time/ [Accessed on 2024-11-14].

12. Estes C. Rwanda Fights Cervical Cancer with Information. *Bio News*, May 24, 2022. Available from: https://bio.news/health/rwanda-fights-cervical-cancer-with-information/ [Accessed on 2024-11-14].

13. Irabor OC, Swanson W, Shaukat F, Wirtz J, Mallum AA, Ngoma T, Elzawawy A, Nguyen P, Incrocci L, Ngwa W. Can the Adoption of Hypofractionation Guidelines Expand Global Radiotherapy Access? An Analysis for Breast and Prostate Radiotherapy. *JCO Glob Oncol.* 2020 Apr;6:667–678.

CHAPTER 6

Sustainability in Global Collaborations

Alfredo Polo, Godfrey Azangwe, Lisbeth Cordero Mendez, Egor Titovich, and Jacob Van Dyk

6.1 CHAPTER OBJECTIVES

- To define sustainability
- To describe factors affecting sustainability
  - Contextual factors
  - Programme factors
- To describe sustainability framework
- To address sustainability metrics and assessment
- To provide recommendations specific to sustainability in global medical physics collaborations

6.2 DEFINITION OF SUSTAINABILITY

When we think of sustainability, especially in the healthcare context and in the developing world, our naive thoughts immediately consider initiatives that get started and continue indefinitely without interruptions, with expected defined and positive outcomes. These simplistic thoughts contain two components: "expected outcome" and "continuity."

DOI: 10.1201/9781003527749-6

Various scholarly articles have attempted to define sustainability, but in many cases, the definitions are based on specific contexts or perspectives. Urquhart *et al.*, when discussing the implementation of real-world innovations in healthcare [1], indicate that "One of the key conceptual challenges in advancing our understanding of how to more effectively sustain innovations is the lack of clarity and agreement on what sustainability actually means." Another broadly based article describes the three pillars of sustainability [2] encompassing economic, social, and environmental (or ecological) factors or goals. Moore *et al.* [3] developed a comprehensive definition of sustainability based on a scoping review, identifying five constructs that relate to time, continued programme delivery, behavioural change and its evolution, and continued benefits.

Others have looked at sustainability in the context of evidence-based health interventions in clinical community settings [4, 5]. Collectively, these definitions converge on continuity, adaptability, and measurable outcomes, highlighting the dynamic nature of sustainability. While Moore *et al.* [3] emphasize adaptation and continuous benefit, Sarriot and Hobson [6] highlight the critical distinction between forward-looking potential (sustainability) and after-the-fact measurement (sustainment). To quote:

- "*Prospectively* – Sustainability refers to the ability, or potential of an entity (local system, health system, organization, etc.) to maintain a function or public good.

- *Retrospectively* – Sustainment refers to the verifiable extent to which a public good has measurably evolved over a time" [6].

Note the difference between *sustainability* and *sustainment*. They define a *sustainment index* as a metric for sustainability in which they measure how the trend of health indicator Y from time $T0$ to time $T1$ continues from time $T1$ to $T2$ (Figure 6.1).

The sustainment index, $SI(Y)$, is defined as

$$SI(Y) = 1 + \left(\frac{YT1 - YT2}{YT0 - YT1} \right)$$

An $SI = 1$ indicates that there is no change in the health indicator; an $SI > 1$ indicates a positive change; and an $SI \leq 1$ indicates a negative change. Note that the SI is a measure of the relative change in the health indicator but does not address the significance or the quality of that health indicator.

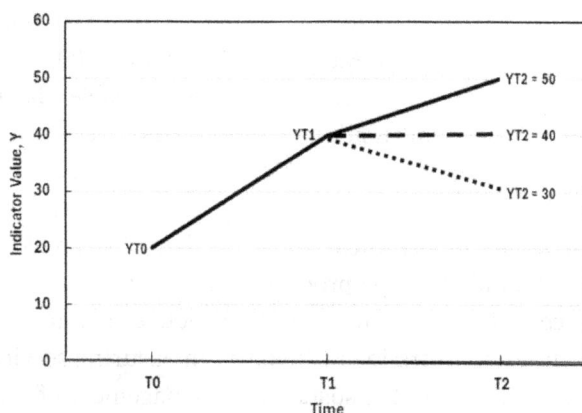

FIGURE 6.1 Three examples of health indicator progress through three points in time (adapted with permission from [6]).

The *SI* tool has several considerations: (1) It identifies the concepts associated with sustainability, i.e., quantification of health indicator and continuity. (2) It encourages quantification of the health indicator. (3) It requires a quantitative measure of health indicator as a function of time. The challenge is determining the appropriate and quantifiable measures of the healthcare indicators for initiatives to be assessed and then to assess them at several well-defined points in time. As an example, Buffoli *et al.* [7] developed specific sustainability metrics for assessing hospitals, taking into consideration the three pillars of sustainability.

6.3 DIMENSIONS OF SUSTAINABILITY

Through a structured literature review, Bodkin *et al.* [8] examined the health promotion programmes (HPP) to see if they maintained their intended benefits from a community capacity perspective and the perspective of financial resources. The review, which included 16 relevant papers, identified 14 key factors influencing programme sustainability: organizational capacity, partnerships, strategic planning, funding stability, fit/alignment by partner organizations, programme monitoring and evaluation, capacity building to allow sustainability, programme champion advocating for the project, communications regarding programme outcomes, programme implementation involving major partners, political support ensuring funding stability, programme adaptation to adjust to local circumstances, public health impacts being actively promoted, and adapting to socio-economic/political factors as they change.

Several factors are essential for sustaining radiotherapy operations, as identified in the joint World Health Organization (WHO)–International Atomic Energy Agency (IAEA) publication, "Sustainable Management of Radiotherapy Facilities and Equipment" [9]. These include robust management support, a well-trained workforce, properly maintained facility infrastructure, and reliable radiotherapy equipment. The document highlights that the failure of any of these critical elements can jeopardize the sustainability of a radiotherapy programme. The publication emphasizes the importance of both preventive and corrective maintenance; details the responsibilities of professionals involved in ensuring service continuity; and offers guidance on the sustainable management of radiotherapy equipment and facilities. This includes processes from procurement to the eventual replacement of equipment, ensuring the long-term functionality and efficiency of radiotherapy programmes.

Sustainability factors can be broadly categorized into two main groups: contextual factors, which reflect the influence of present conditions and local circumstances, and programmatic factors, which pertain to organizational dynamics [10]. These categories provide a framework for understanding the diverse elements that affect sustainability. Figure 6.2 summarizes these two components, showing significant overlap with the factors identified before by Bodkin *et al.* [8] and the WHO/IAEA joint

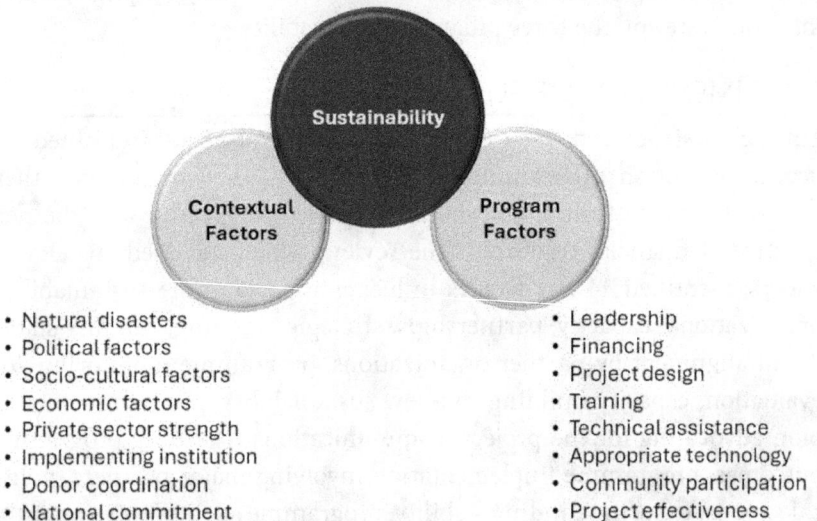

- Natural disasters
- Political factors
- Socio-cultural factors
- Economic factors
- Private sector strength
- Implementing institution
- Donor coordination
- National commitment

- Leadership
- Financing
- Project design
- Training
- Technical assistance
- Appropriate technology
- Community participation
- Project effectiveness

FIGURE 6.2 Examples of sustainability factors as divided into contextual and programmatic contexts.

publication. This alignment underscores the interconnectedness of local contexts and organizational strategies in shaping the long-term viability of programmes.

6.4 SUSTAINABILITY FRAMEWORK

The Washington University in St Louis has developed a sustainability framework, which identifies a small set of organizational and contextual domains that help build the capacity for maintaining a programme. They define sustainability capacity as the ability to maintain programming and its benefits over time. The sustainability capacity involves eight key domains that can influence a programme's capacity. These are summarized in Figure 6.3. Along with the domains, they have developed the Programme Sustainability Assessment Tool (PSAT), which can be used to guide sustainability action planning for that programme. Local (hospital) administrators and medical physicists can collaboratively score these eight domains, prioritize gaps, and develop targeted action plans for improving sustainability capacity using a commercial PSAT.

Program Sustainability Framework and Domain Descriptions v3

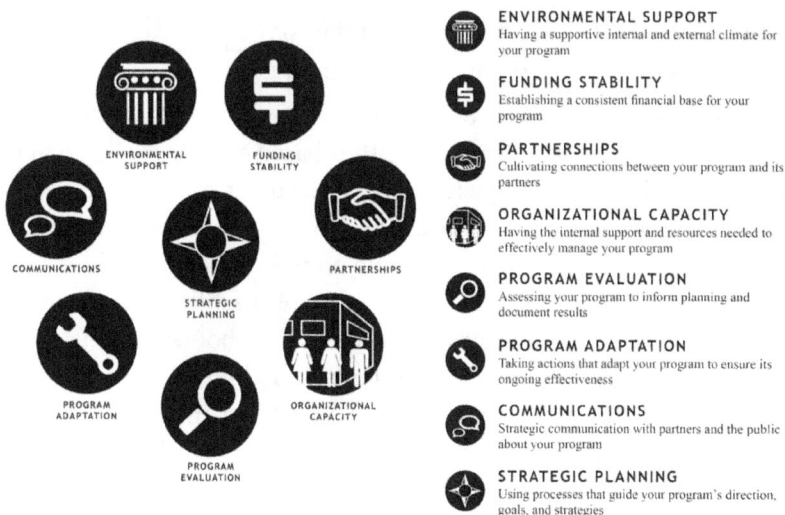

FIGURE 6.3   Eight key domains that influence a program's capacity for sustainability (adapted with permission from [11]).

6.5 INDICES HIGHLIGHTING POTENTIAL BARRIERS TO SUSTAINABILITY

Sustainability in healthcare programmes depends on a thorough understanding of the contextual factors that influence their success or failure. Indices such as gross domestic product (GDP) [12], gross national income (GNI) [13], and human development index (HDI) [14] offer critical insights into a country's economic and social landscape, while metrics like the Hassle Factor (HF) [15] and Corruption Perceptions Index (CPI) [16] reveal logistical and governance-related challenges. These tools are not just indicators of potential barriers; they are essential for informed decision-making. By analyzing these indices, stakeholders can pinpoint areas of vulnerability, allocate resources strategically, and design interventions tailored to the specific needs of each context. While these indices guide initial feasibility assessments, project-specific metrics – like equipment uptime or local workforce stability – remain critical for a granular understanding of barriers on the ground.

Note that this is not an exhaustive list of indices. For example, there is a list of *freedom* indices ranking countries at several levels of freedom, using various measures of freedom, including civil liberties, political rights, and economic rights [17]. Another is the *Ease of Doing Business* as described by the World Bank Group [18].

6.6 SUSTAINABILITY OF RADIOTHERAPY IN AFRICA

6.6.1 Accessibility Considerations for Radiotherapy

Figure 6.4 shows the number of operational megavoltage radiation therapy machines installed in Africa since 1991 based on data available in the IAEA DIRAC database along with some of the descriptive indices.

The darker shade shows countries where the number of machines declined from some level to zero at some point in time. The lighter shade shows countries where a significant number of machines have provided ongoing clinical service. The averages shown at the bottom for the darker and lighter categories clearly show some trends although these have not been tested statistically, nor should these data be over-interpreted. To reiterate, they just contribute to the total background knowledge related to specific attributes of those countries.

Clearly, there are many other, perhaps more important, factors in assessing whether a new initiative will be successful and sustainable. In some countries, there is an initial investment to acquire a radiotherapy

Country Name	1991	1997	2000	2010	2013	2015	2018	2020	2023	GDP/capita (2022)	GNI/capita (2022)	HDI (2022)	HF (2018)	CPI (2023)
Algeria	4	23	23	17	19	19	38	37	55	$ 11,758	$ 11,479	0.75	4.48	36
Angola	0	1	1	1	3	3	3	3	3	$ 6,201	$ 5,655	0.59	5.40	33
Botswana	0	0	0	1	1	1	1	1	2	$ 16,295	$ 15,754	0.71	3.53	59
Burkina Faso	0	0	0	0	0	0	0	0	4	$ 2,267	$ -	0.44	5.50	41
Cameroon	3	2	2	2	1	1	1	1	2	$ 3,910	$ 3,850	0.59	4.82	27
Congo, Democratic Republic of the	1	0	0	1	0	0	0	0	2	$ 1,838	$ 1,127	0.48	5.60	20
Congo, Republic of the	1	1	0	0	0	0	0	0	0	$ 3,854	$ 3,646	0.59	5.16	22
Cote D'Ivoire	0	0	0	0	0	0	0	2	2	$ 5,814	$ 5,645	0.53	4.90	40
Egypt	31	23	23	55	74	67	119	117	122	$ 13,420	$ 12,978	0.73	3.80	35
Ethiopia	0	1	1	3	2	2	2	2	7	$ 2,500	$ 2,489	0.49	5.09	37
Gabon	1	0	0	1	2	2	3	2	2	$ 14,637	$ 11,744	0.69	4.63	28
Ghana	0	2	2	2	3	5	4	5	5	$ 5,754	$ 5,678	0.60	3.88	43
Kenya	2	3	3	5	6	8	11	12	17	$ 5,126	$ 5,048	0.60	4.10	31
Libya	1	5	5	8	4	3	3	6	6	$ 20,787	$ 25,681	0.75	5.08	18
Madagascar	1	1	1	1	1	3	2	2	3	$ 1,577	$ 1,538	0.49	4.74	25
Mali	0	0	0	0	0	1	1	1	1	$ 2,240	$ 2,147	0.41	5.10	28
Mauritania	0	0	0	1	1	1	1	2	2	$ 5,597	$ 5,559	0.54	5.32	30
Mauritius	1	4	4	3	3	3	3	3	4	$ 23,983	$ 23,537	0.80	3.01	50
Morocco	3	7	7	14	30	33	38	42	66	$ 8,487	$ 8,373	0.70	3.65	38
Mozambique	0	1	1	0	0	0	0	1	1	$ 1,314	$ 1,264	0.46	4.59	25
Namibia	0	1	1	1	1	2	2	2	3	$ 10,251	$ 9,930	0.61	3.64	49
Niger	0	0	0	0	0	0	0	0	1	$ 1,339	$ 1,347	0.39		32
Nigeria	2	5	5	4	13	13	2	7	8	$ 5,211	$ 4,952	0.55	5.22	25
Rwanda	0	0	0	0	0	0	0	2	2	$ 2,483	$ 2,433	0.55	4.33	53
Senegal	0	1	1	2	1	1	4	3	3	$ 3,743	$ 3,605	0.52	4.69	43
South Africa	0	47	47	60	76	81	93	103	106	$ 14,153	$ 14,198	0.72	3.06	41
Sudan	2	4	4	5	10	8	8	10	10	$ 3,750	$ 3,691	0.52	5.19	20
Tanzania	2	1	1	3	3	2	6	5	7	$ 2,755	$ 2,708	0.53	5.04	40
Togo	0	0	0	0	0	0	0	0	1	$ 2,313	$ 2,317	0.55	5.37	31
Tunisia	3	7	7	11	15	19	22	24	24	$ 11,097	$ 10,815	0.73	4.62	40
Uganda	0	2	2	1	1	1	1	1	5	$ 2,394	$ 2,346	0.55	4.59	26
Zambia	0	0	0	2	3	2	3	3	0	$ 3,534	$ 3,407	0.57	4.71	37
Zimbabwe	4	5	5	3	3	4	6	7	1	$ 2,318	$ 2,251	0.55	4.53	24
Total	62			276		377			477					
Average										$ 3,140	$ 2,928	0.54	4.95	26
Average										$ 10,674	$ 10,482	0.70	3.95	37

Countries with sustained radiotherapy
Countries without sustained radiotherapy

FIGURE 6.4   Radiotherapy machines installed in Africa since 1991 along with some of the descriptive indices for those countries. The averages show the mean values of those highlighted in dark shade (not sustained) and light shade (sustained). GDP/capita, https://ourworldindata.org/grapher/gdp-per-capita-world-bank?tab=table; GNI/capita, https://ourworldindata.org/grapher/gross-national-income-per-capita; HDI, https://en.wikipedia.org/wiki/List_of_countries_by_Human_Development_Index; HF, https://www.ivey.uwo.ca/internationalbusiness/research/hasslefactor/rankings/2018/; CPI, https://www.transparency.org/en/cpi/2023.

machine without adequate planning for maintenance and service contracts. In other cases, the cost of maintaining the service contracts competes with other country's priorities, resulting in contracts being stopped. In low- and middle-income countries (LMICs), another challenge is the brain drain of skilled professionals such as medical physicists, radiation oncologists, radiation therapists, and electronics service personnel affecting consistent service delivery. The WHO in collaboration with the IAEA has provided some recommendations in their publication on sustainable management of radiotherapy facilities and equipment [9].

Sustaining operations in the radiotherapy chain presents several challenges. In brief, the challenges include:

- Lack of long-term financial commitment to ensure the continuity of services after the initial procurement.

- Lack of strategic planning when considering the whole equipment life cycle from initial procurement to replacement.

- Service contracts are often handled by third-party service companies who charge exorbitant margins compared to what the equipment vendors charge in other regions.

- Considerations of facility infrastructure maintenance such as air conditioning, water, and power supply necessary to operate the devices in the radiotherapy equipment chain.

- Enablement of robust data sharing within regional (or international) networks to help track machine downtime, to identify trends in equipment failures, and to pinpoint precisely where targeted financial or workforce interventions are needed.

6.6.2 UN-Led Initiatives in Cancer Control

On a much broader scale, a prime example of detailed preparatory assessments for developments of national cancer control programmes in LMICs is described by Veljkovikj *et al.* [19]. The WHO, International Agency for Cancer Research (IARC), and IAEA collaborate through imPACT reviews to advise and support LMICs in developing sustainable cancer control. Political and financial commitments, alongside thorough assessments, are key to sustaining long-term progress. These high-level reviews need to be paired with robust data-capture methods, ensuring that policy decisions are anchored in empirical evidence.

6.7 A MULTI-SECTORAL APPROACH TO SUSTAINABILITY

Sustainability in medical physics cannot be achieved through isolated efforts. A multi-sectoral approach is essential, integrating contributions from research, clinical services, education, and workforce development to address complex challenges and ensure long-term impact across all dimensions of care.

6.7.1 Research

Research fosters innovation and continuous improvement [20] with activities varying according to locally available resources and the research network within the country. Examples include IAEA's Coordinated Research

Program, including clinical trials, with collaborative efforts from both LMICs and HICs.

6.7.2 Clinical Service

The medical physics service available in a country relates directly to the need for the service, which, of course, relates to the relevant imaging and radiotherapy technologies available in a department, region, or country. If there are no machines/technologies in a country, then there is no need for medical physicists. If we look at the data of Figure 6.4, the sustainability of medical physics needs goes down dramatically when there are no radiation therapy machines in the country.

6.7.3 Education

Moreland-Russell *et al.* [4] have developed a conceptual model for building programme sustainability in public health settings. While their paper presents the results of a sustainability training intervention and a conceptual model of sustainability in another context, participants found intervention components (workshop, workbook, instructor, and resources) to be effective.

6.7.4 Sustainability through Decent Jobs

A sustainable medical physics programme requires not only robust infrastructure but also a well-supported workforce. Decent jobs are central to sustainability by ensuring fair compensation, job security, and professional growth for medical physicists and related professionals. Key barriers in LMICs include brain drain, limited career opportunities, inadequate working conditions, and lack of professional recognition, which hinder retention and motivation. Quantitative tracking of staff retention, job satisfaction, and training outcomes can demonstrate the return on investment for local governments, creating an evidence-based argument for continuing to fund decent jobs. Promoting incentives for local talent retention, offering continuous professional development, and fostering better policies to create and sustain decent jobs are essential. These policies (e.g., workforce planning, labour rights, or funding mechanisms) should prioritize fair labour practices, ensure equitable compensation, and provide structured career pathways. Partnerships with international organizations can further support the development of a skilled and motivated workforce.

6.8 SUSTAINABILITY INDICATORS AND ASSESSMENT

Ideally, for every global health project, the success of the programme would be assessed by evaluating the outcome of specific sustainability indicators. Waas *et al.* [21] describe sustainable assessment and sustainable indicators as tools for decision-making strategies for sustainable development. They highlight the fundamental elements of any sustainable assessment and sustainable indicator, i.e., (1) interpreting sustainability; (2) measuring and understanding the success of the sustainability indicators; and (3) exerting influence on decision-making in support of sustainable development. The application of the sustainability index aids in the quantification of the success of the project.

6.9 SUMMARY AND RECOMMENDATIONS

6.9.1 Summary

Sustainable programmes in the context of global health initiatives especially as related to medical physics involve several key concepts: (1) continuity for a defined period of time, (2) successful implementation of strategies for improvement, (3) successful education programmes resulting in change of practice for enhancements in patient treatments, and (4) well-defined metrics to determine the success of the programme. There are multiple factors involved in developing successful and sustainable programmes, which can be loosely categorized as contextual and programmatic factors. Contextual factors involve the three pillars of sustainability including economic, social, and environmental considerations. The programmatic factors relate to the direct activities of the programme ranging from leadership to financing, to training, and to appropriate technology. Eight key domains have been defined that influence a programme's capacity for sustainability: environmental support, funding stability, equal partnerships, organizational capacity, programme evaluation, programme adaptation, communication, and strategic planning. Various indices are available that relate to a country's economic status as well as allowing for an assessment of potential barriers to successful development projects. The sustainability considerations described in this chapter provide an overall framework that is useful for project decision-makers as well as those who are directly involved in organizing and/or implementing such projects.

6.9.2 Recommendations and Points of Interest

1. The implementation of successful and sustainable projects begins with a well-designed plan and is implemented with the following broad considerations:

(a) organizational capacity to effectively manage the project

(b) strong partnerships

(c) strategic planning providing programme direction

(d) funding stability

(e) fit/alignment by partner organizations

(f) programme monitoring and evaluation

(g) capacity building to allow sustainability

(h) a programme champion advocating for the project

(i) communications regarding programme outcomes

(j) programme implementation involving major partners

(k) political support ensuring funding stability

(l) programme adaptation to adjust to contemporary circumstances

(m) public health impacts being actively promoted

(n) adapting to socio-economic/political factors as they change

2. Specifically, a new project or programme requires:

(a) Assessment that evaluates the specific medical physics needs of the region, taking into account demographics, culture, health practices, available technologies along with their maintenance programmes, and overall infrastructure.

(b) Engagement with local stakeholders (e.g., healthcare leaders, medical physicists, and other relevant healthcare workers) in this process to ensure the programme is tailored to local needs and has direct local involvement from the start.

(c) Understanding of the local health system to identify gaps in healthcare infrastructure, workforce capacity, and essential services, thus enabling targeted improvements.

(d) Multi-sector collaboration with government health agencies, NGOs, local businesses, and academic institutions to leverage shared resources, knowledge, and expertise.

3. Use a sustainability evaluation tool as part of the planning process for a new global health project.

REFERENCES

1. Urquhart, R., *et al.*, Defining sustainability in practice: views from implementing real-world innovations in health care. *BMC Health Serv Res*, 2020. **20**(1): p. 87.
2. Purvis, B., Y. Mao, and D. Robinson, Three pillars of sustainability: in search of conceptual origins. *Sust Sci*, 2019. **14**: p. 681–695.
3. Moore, J.E., *et al.*, Developing a comprehensive definition of sustainability. *Implement Sci*, 2017. **12**(1): p. 110.
4. Moreland-Russell, S., E. Jost, and J. Gannon, A conceptual model for building program sustainability in public health settings: learning from the implementation of the program sustainability action planning model and training curricula. *Front Health Serv*, 2023. **3**: p. 1026484.
5. Johnson, A.M., *et al.*, How do researchers conceptualize and plan for the sustainability of their NIH R01 implementation projects? *Implement Sci*, 2019. **14**(1): p. 50.
6. Sarriot, E. and R.D. Hobson, A simple metric for a complex outcome: proposing a sustainment index for health indicators. *BMC Health Serv Res*, 2018. **18**(1): p. 538.
7. Buffoli, M., et al., Sustainable healthcare: how to assess and improve healthcare structures' sustainability. *Ann Ig*, 2013. **25**(5): p. 411–418.
8. Bodkin, A. and S. Hakimi, Sustainable by design: a systematic review of factors for health promotion program sustainability. *BMC Public Health*, 2020. **20**(1): p. 964.
9. World Health Organization (WHO). Sustainable Management of Radiotherapy Facilities and Equipment. 2023; Available from: https://www.are.admin.ch/are/en/home/media/publications/sustainable-development/brundtland-report.html [Accessed 2024-12-14].
10. Thuo, I.W., K. Ndiaye, and S. Mookherji, Factors influencing the sustainability of neglected tropical disease elimination programs: a multi-case study of the Kenya National Program for Elimination of Lymphatic Filariasis. *Am J Trop Med Hyg*, 2020. **102**(5): p. 1090–1093.
11. Center for Public Health Systems Science, W.U., ST. Louis, MO, Program sustainability assessment tool. 2023; Available from: https://sustaintool.org/psat/understand/ [Accesssed 2025-02-14].
12. Our World Data. GDP per capita. 2024; Available from: https://ourworldindata.org/grapher/gdp-per-capita-worldbank?tab=table [Accessed 2024-12-14].
13. Our World Data. GNI per capita. 2024; Available from: https://ourworldindata.org/grapher/gross-national-income-per-capita [Accessed 2024-12-14].
14. United Nations Development Program. Human development index (HDI). 2024; Available from: https://hdr.undp.org/data-center/human-development-index#/indicies/HDI [Accessed 2024-12-14].

15. Ivey Business School. The hassle factor. Available from: https://www.ivey
    .uwo.ca/internationalbusiness/research/hasslefactor/ [Accessed 2025-01-
    14].
16. Transparency International. Corruption perceptions index. 2024; Available
    from: https://www.transparency.org/en/cpi/2023 [Accessed 2024-12-15].
17. Wikipedia. List of Freedom Indices. 2024; Available from: https://en.wiki-
    pedia.org/wiki/List_of_freedom_indices [Accessed 2024-12-15].
18. World Bank Group. Ease of doing business rankings. 2024; Available from:
    https://archive.doingbusiness.org/en/rankings [Accessed 2024-12-15].
19. Veljkovikj, I., *et al.*, Evolution of the joint International Atomic Energy
    Agency (IAEA), International Agency for Research on Cancer (IARC), and
    WHO cancer control assessments (imPACT Reviews). *Lancet Oncol*, 2022.
    23(10): p. e459–e468.
20. Abdel-Wahab, M., *et al.*, Global radiotherapy: current status and future
    directions: White Paper. *JCO Glob Oncol*, 2021. 7: p. 827–842.
21. Waas, T., *et al.*, Sustainability assessment and indicators: tools in a decision-
    making strategy for sustainable development. *Sustainability*, 2014. **6**(9): p.
    5512–5534.

CHAPTER 7

Career Paths in Medical Physics with a Global Health Perspective

Stephen M. Avery

7.1 CHAPTER OBJECTIVES

- To describe the various career paths available to medical physicists
- For each career path, to describe
  - Core responsibilities
  - Education and training requirements
  - Contributions to global health
  - Challenges and opportunities
- To describe global health initiatives and how medical physicists can contribute to them
- To provide a summary and suggestions on how medical physicists can be involved in global health initiatives

7.2 INTRODUCTION

Medical physics is an interdisciplinary field that applies physics principles to medicine, with the primary goal of improving healthcare outcomes.

DOI: 10.1201/9781003527749-7

TABLE 7.1   Overview of Career Paths in Medical Physics with Corresponding Education Requirements

Career Path	Education Requirements
Clinical practice	PhD or master's degree + Residency + Certification (e.g., ABR, IMPCB)
Academia	PhD in medical physics or related field + Research and teaching experience
Research	PhD + Postdoctoral training + Specialized skills (e.g., AI, nanotechnology)
Industry	Master's or PhD + Knowledge of regulations (e.g., FDA, CE Marking)
Global health initiatives	Master's or PhD + Cultural competence + Public health training

Medical physicists contribute to diverse areas, including diagnostic imaging, radiation therapy, and nuclear medicine, making them critical in advancing global health. With cancer being a leading cause of death worldwide, the expertise of medical physicists is particularly vital in improving the availability and quality of radiation-based diagnosis and treatment.

Global health initiatives have highlighted the disparity in healthcare resources, particularly in LMICs where access to advanced medical technologies is limited. Medical physicists can address these challenges through various career paths. This chapter explores five major career options – *Clinical Practice, Academia, Research, Industry,* and *Global Health Initiatives* – detailing the roles, educational requirements, skills, and contributions to global health (Table 7.1). By understanding these paths, aspiring medical physicists can align their careers to meet both professional goals and global healthcare needs.

7.3 CLINICAL PRACTICE

Clinical practice forms the foundation of medical physics, where professionals apply physics principles in healthcare to ensure the safe and effective use of radiation for diagnosis and treatment. Clinical medical physicists collaborate with radiation oncologists, radiologists, and healthcare teams to deliver high-quality patient care. Their multifaceted role includes technical oversight, operational management, safety assurance, and training, which are critical to healthcare systems worldwide.

7.3.1 Core Responsibilities

Clinical medical physicists perform tasks aimed at optimizing patient safety and treatment efficacy:

1. **Quality Assurance (QA):**

   - Regular testing, calibration, and maintenance of equipment, such as linear accelerators and CT scanners, ensure peak performance and prevent errors that could compromise patient safety.

2. **Dosimetry:**

   - Precise radiation dose calculations, developed in collaboration with oncologists, maximize tumour targeting while minimizing harm to healthy tissues.

3. **Protocol Development:**

   - Establishing standardized procedures ensures consistent, safe, and regulation-compliant radiation use across treatment settings.

4. **Incident Management:**

   - Investigating equipment malfunctions or deviations in radiation delivery ensures rapid resolution and prevents recurrence, safeguarding patient outcomes.

5. **Patient-Specific Applications:**

   - Advanced procedures like stereotactic body radiotherapy (SBRT) and proton therapy demand tailored treatment plans for optimal precision and effectiveness.

6. **Training and Mentorship:**

   - Training healthcare professionals in complex diagnostic and therapeutic technologies builds capacity and enhances care delivery, especially in resource-limited settings.

7.3.2 Education and Training Requirements

Becoming a clinical medical physicist requires rigorous academic preparation and practical experience:

1. **Educational Background:**

   - A master's or PhD in Medical Physics provides foundational knowledge in radiation physics, imaging, and treatment planning. Accredited programmes, such as CAMPEP [1], ensure comprehensive training.

2. **Clinical Training:**

- Residency programmes offer hands-on experience in QA, dosimetry, and patient care, bridging academic knowledge with real-world application.

3. **Certification Requirements:**

- Certifications from organizations like the American Board of Radiology (ABR) or the International Medical Physics Certification Board (IMPCB) validate expertise. Ongoing professional development ensures physicists stay updated with evolving technologies and best practices [2, 3].

7.3.3 Contributions to Global Health

Clinical physicists are pivotal in addressing global health disparities, particularly in LMICs:

1. **Expanding Access:**

- Collaborating with organizations like the International Atomic Energy Agency (IAEA), physicists design and implement radiotherapy facilities in underserved regions [4].

2. **Capacity Building:**

- Training programmes and mentorship initiatives empower local healthcare workers, fostering sustainable healthcare systems.

3. **Patient Safety:**

- Implementing QA protocols and optimizing treatment plans minimize risks and improve care quality.

4. **Collaboration:**

- Initiatives like the IAEA's *Rays of Hope* expand access to essential technologies in LMICs [5].

7.3.4 Challenges and Opportunities

Clinical practice faces challenges, including infrastructure deficiencies, workforce shortages, and sustainability concerns. However, emerging technologies like AI-driven treatment planning and MR-guided radiotherapy, coupled with global collaborations, provide opportunities for significant impact. Leadership roles enable experienced physicists to shape cancer care policies and protocols on national and international levels.

Clinical practice is the cornerstone of medical physics, ensuring patient safety, fostering innovation, and promoting equitable healthcare. Clinical physicists' expertise is crucial for addressing global health disparities and advancing cancer care worldwide.

7.4 ACADEMIA

Academia is a cornerstone of medical physics, where professionals engage in education, research, and leadership to advance the field. Academic medical physicists shape the future of healthcare by training the next generation, conducting innovative research, and advocating for equity in access to medical services. In global health, their work addresses disparities in access and quality of care while fostering sustainable healthcare systems.

7.4.1 Roles and Responsibilities

Academic medical physicists play multifaceted roles as educators, researchers, mentors, and leaders, influencing healthcare systems at local and global levels:

1. **Teaching:**

   - Academic physicists deliver comprehensive courses covering radiobiology, imaging modalities, and radiation therapy. Leveraging innovative tools like virtual simulations and online platforms, they enhance accessibility, particularly in underserved regions.

2. **Mentorship:**

   - Guiding students, residents, and early-career professionals is crucial, especially in LMICs, where mentorship helps nurture local talent and build self-reliant healthcare systems. (See Chapter 8 on Mentoring in the Global Context.)

3. **Research:**

   - Academics lead studies to develop novel technologies and optimize existing ones. Research often focuses on global health priorities, such as cost-effective radiotherapy protocols for resource-limited settings.

4. **Leadership:**

- Academic physicists manage departments, design curricula, and lead institutional initiatives that align educational goals with healthcare needs. These roles promote interdisciplinary collaboration and institutional growth.

5. **Global Health Advocacy:**

- Collaborating with organizations like the IAEA and the World Health Organization (WHO), academic medical physicists develop training programmes tailored to underserved regions and advocate for equitable healthcare policies [6]. (See Chapter 11 on Advocacy and Science Diplomacy.)

7.4.2 Education and Training Requirements

A career in academia requires a combination of advanced education, research experience, and teaching skills:

1. **PhD in Medical Physics or Related Fields:**

- A doctoral degree equips candidates with the expertise needed for tenure-track positions, independent research, and advanced teaching roles.

2. **Research Experience:**

- Demonstrated competency through peer-reviewed publications, conference presentations, and interdisciplinary projects is essential.

3. **Teaching Competence:**

- Experience gained through teaching assistantships or workshops provides a foundation. Certifications in pedagogy enhance effectiveness in diverse educational settings.

4. **Global Health Training:**

- Additional training in public health or cultural competence prepares academics for international collaborations and global health-focused initiatives [7].

7.4.3 Contributions to Global Health

Academic medical physicists play a transformative role in addressing global health challenges:

1. **Developing Education Programmes:**

   - Curricula tailored to the challenges of LMICs focus on affordability, sustainability, and accessibility. Distance learning platforms extend the reach of education to underserved regions.

2. **Knowledge Exchange:**

   - Collaborations between institutions in high-income and low-income countries facilitate mutual growth and resource sharing.

3. **Advancing Global Health Research:**

   - Research targeting diseases prevalent in LMICs, such as cervical and breast cancer, leads to affordable and effective diagnostic and therapeutic tools.

4. **Building Local Capacity:**

   - Partnerships with local institutions help establish medical physics programmes, train faculty, and create sustainable educational models.

5. **Policy Advocacy:**

   - Academic research provides evidence-based recommendations that inform healthcare policies and strategies [8].

7.4.4 Challenges

Despite its contributions, academia faces challenges that complicate its global health impact:

1. **Funding Limitations:**

   - Long-term global health projects struggle to secure funding, as grants often prioritize short-term outcomes.

2. **Resource Inequities:**

- Institutions in LMICs frequently lack adequate teaching materials, laboratories, and access to current research publications.

3. **Brain Drain:**

- Trained professionals often migrate to high-income countries, reducing the local impact of academic programmes [9].

4. **Balancing Roles:**

- Managing teaching, research, and administrative responsibilities can be demanding, especially in global collaborations.

5. **Cultural Barriers:**

- Overcoming linguistic and cultural differences is necessary for effective programme implementation [10].

7.4.5 Opportunities for Growth

Academia offers substantial opportunities for innovation and global impact:

1. **Interdisciplinary Research:**

- Collaborations with engineers, data scientists, and clinicians drive advancements in AI-based diagnostics and adaptive radiotherapy techniques.

2. **Global Collaborations:**

- Partnerships with international organizations provide platforms for addressing large-scale global health challenges.

3. **Educational Technology:**

- Tools like virtual reality (VR) and augmented reality (AR) revolutionize medical physics education, enabling immersive learning experiences.

4. **Leadership Roles:**

- Academic physicists often ascend to leadership positions, influencing institutional growth and the future of the field.

5. **Influential Publications:**

- High-impact research reaches broad audiences, shaping policies and practices in medical physics and healthcare.

7.5 RESEARCH

Research in medical physics is a driving force behind innovation, advancing diagnostic and therapeutic technologies to improve healthcare outcomes. Medical physicists bridge theoretical science and clinical application, focusing on affordability, accessibility, and sustainability. Their contributions are critical in addressing healthcare disparities, particularly in low- and middle-income countries (LMICs), where access to advanced technologies remains limited [11].

7.5.1 Core Responsibilities

Research physicists in medical physics take on diverse roles to innovate and optimize healthcare technologies:

1. **Developing New Technologies:**

- They contribute to innovations like proton therapy systems and adaptive radiotherapy techniques, enhancing precision and effectiveness in cancer treatment.

- In LMICs, research focuses on cost-effective solutions, such as portable imaging devices and simplified radiotherapy systems.

2. **Optimizing Existing Technologies:**

- Researchers improve the efficiency and usability of existing equipment by enhancing imaging resolution, reducing radiation exposure, and increasing system reliability.

3. **Radiation Safety Studies:**

- Investigating the biological effects of radiation helps develop safer dosimetry protocols, vital for patient and worker safety, especially in LMICs with limited regulatory oversight.

4. AI and Machine Learning Applications:

- AI tools enable faster image analysis, predictive modelling, and treatment planning, with adaptations for use in resource-constrained environments [12].

5. Collaborative Projects:

- Interdisciplinary collaboration with engineers, biologists, and clinicians ensures the translation of research into practical, impactful healthcare solutions.

6. Global Health Initiatives:

- Researchers address the unique challenges of LMICs by designing sustainable and culturally appropriate technologies.

7.5.2 Education and Training Requirements

Becoming a research physicist involves advanced education and specialized training:

1. PhD in Medical Physics or Related Fields:

- A doctoral degree combines coursework in imaging, radiation therapy, and computational modelling with hands-on research, preparing physicists to lead independent projects.

2. Postdoctoral Fellowships:

- Fellowships offer specialization in cutting-edge fields like nanotechnology and AI, fostering professional networks and grant-funded experience.

3. Technical Skills:

- Proficiency in programming languages (e.g., Python, MATLAB) and simulation tools is essential for innovation and data analysis.

4. Global Health Training:

- Training in public health equips researchers to design solutions tailored to the unique needs of LMICs.

7.5.3 Contributions to Global Health

Research physicists address global health challenges by:

1. **Developing Affordable Technologies:**

   - Creating tools like portable ultrasound devices and low-cost linear accelerators improves access to essential diagnostics and treatments.

2. **Advancing AI Applications:**

   - AI-driven tools assist in early detection and personalized treatment planning, particularly in areas lacking trained specialists.

3. **Enhancing Radiation Safety:**

   - Improved safety protocols reduce unnecessary radiation exposure, benefiting patients and healthcare workers alike.

4. **Collaborating with Global Organizations:**

   - Partnerships with entities like the IAEA and WHO ensure innovations reach underserved regions.

5. **Addressing Disease Burdens in LMICs:**

   - Research targets high-prevalence diseases such as cervical and breast cancer, improving treatment affordability and accessibility.

7.5.4 Challenges and Opportunities

Despite its promise, research in medical physics faces challenges:

1. **Funding Disparities:**

   - Global health research often struggles to secure adequate funding, limiting the scope of impactful projects [13].

2. **Infrastructure Gaps:**

   - Lack of well-equipped laboratories and reliable resources in LMICs hinders research efforts.

3. **Ethical and Practical Barriers:**

- Ethical considerations, iterative testing, and the translation of technologies into culturally appropriate solutions require significant collaboration and adaptability.

7.6 INDUSTRY

Medical physicists in the industry are essential for bridging the gap between innovation and clinical application, driving the development and dissemination of advanced healthcare technologies. Their contributions span research and development (R&D), regulatory compliance, quality assurance, technical support, and global health initiatives. These professionals ensure technologies are accessible worldwide, with a particular focus on addressing disparities in LMICs [14].

7.6.1 Core Responsibilities

1. **Product Development:**

- Industry physicists collaborate with engineers to design cutting-edge technologies such as adaptive radiotherapy systems, portable imaging devices, and AI-powered diagnostic tools. Innovations are tailored to clinical needs and global safety standards.

- In LMICs, they focus on cost-effective solutions like simplified linear accelerators and energy-efficient devices to address resource constraints.

2. **Regulatory Compliance:**

- Navigating regulatory frameworks ensures product approval by agencies like the US Food and Drug Administration (FDA) and the European Medicines Agency (EMA), enabling international market access and adherence to regional standards [15].

3. **Quality Assurance (QA) and Testing:**

- Physicists establish QA protocols and conduct rigorous testing to ensure devices are safe, effective, and reliable in clinical settings.

4. **Technical Support and Training:**

- Training healthcare providers in the operation and maintenance of equipment ensures sustainability and improved user experience. Feedback is integrated into product refinement.

5. **Research and Innovation:**

- R&D projects focus on creating technologies that prioritize affordability, durability, and sustainability, addressing healthcare challenges specific to LMICs.

6. **Market Expansion:**

- Identifying opportunities to introduce technologies to underserved regions helps tailor solutions to meet local needs.

7.6.2 Contributions to Global Health

Industry physicists play a critical role in improving healthcare access and equity, particularly in underserved areas:

1. **Affordable Technologies:**

- Portable X-ray machines and low-cost brachytherapy systems enhance healthcare delivery in remote regions.

2. **Technology Transfer:**

- Collaborations with governments and NGOs facilitate the deployment of cultural and infrastructure-appropriate technologies.

3. **Training and Support:**

- Building local capacity by training healthcare workers reduces dependence on external expertise and ensures sustainable usage.

4. **Public–Private Partnerships (PPPs):**

- Partnerships subsidize equipment costs and provide long-term maintenance support, making healthcare technologies accessible. (See Chapter 5.)

7.6.3 Challenges and Opportunities

1. **Challenges:**

- Balancing profit with affordability, navigating diverse regulatory frameworks, addressing infrastructure limitations, and ensuring sustainability are ongoing concerns.

2. **Opportunities:**

- Emerging technologies like AI-driven diagnostics and hybrid imaging systems present significant growth opportunities. Expanding into LMIC markets and developing energy-efficient devices offer avenues for impactful innovation.

7.7 GLOBAL HEALTH INITIATIVES

Global health initiatives aim to address disparities in healthcare access, particularly in underserved regions, by improving the availability and quality of critical medical services. Medical physicists play a crucial role in tackling systemic challenges in cancer care and diagnostics, collaborating with international organizations, governments, and NGOs. Their work spans policy advocacy, capacity building, and infrastructure development, fostering sustainable advancements in global healthcare systems [16].

7.7.1 Core Responsibilities

1. **Policy Development and Advocacy:**

- Medical physicists advise governments and global health organizations on strategies to enhance cancer care infrastructure. Their contributions to national cancer control plans (NCCPs) and advocacy for funding ensure expanded access to radiation therapy and diagnostic services.

2. **Capacity Building:**

- Training healthcare professionals, including physicists, radiologists, and technicians, equips local teams to operate and maintain medical equipment sustainably. Mentorship programmes and workshops promote knowledge transfer.

3. **Infrastructure Development:**

- Physicists play a critical role in establishing radiotherapy centres and diagnostic imaging facilities, ensuring proper equipment installation, calibration, and site readiness for safe operations.

4. **Technology Implementation:**

- Developing affordable and durable medical devices tailored to resource-constrained settings, such as portable imaging systems, addresses the unique needs of underserved regions.

5. **International Collaboration:**

- Partnerships with organizations like the IAEA and the WHO drive large-scale initiatives, such as expanding radiotherapy access and improving diagnostic services.

6. **Monitoring and Evaluation:**

- Medical physicists assess global health programmes by measuring outcomes like increased treatment capacity, enhanced patient safety, and improved workforce competency.

7.7.2 Contributions to Global Health

Medical physicists significantly impact global health through their technical expertise and advocacy:

1. **Addressing the Global Cancer Burden:**

- Initiatives like the IAEA's *Rays of Hope* establish radiotherapy facilities in LMICs, closing treatment gaps and reducing cancer mortality rates.

2. **Building Sustainable Systems:**

- Developing quality assurance protocols, training local professionals, and designing low-maintenance technologies foster self-reliant healthcare systems.

3. **Technology Transfer:**

- Collaborating with manufacturers ensures that affordable, effective technologies are tailored to the needs of underserved regions.

4. **Strengthening Education:**

- Academic partnerships, such as the African Regional Cooperative Agreement for Research, Development, and Training (AFRA) [17], build a skilled workforce for LMICs.

7.7.3 Challenges and Opportunities

1. **Challenges:**

   - Limited funding, workforce shortages, and logistical barriers complicate the implementation of sustainable healthcare solutions in LMICs. Political and cultural barriers further hinder progress.

2. **Opportunities:**

   - Innovations in AI, telemedicine, and portable devices offer tools for addressing disparities. Expanding collaborations with global organizations and focusing on preventative care create scalable and impactful interventions.

7.8 SUMMARY AND OPPORTUNITIES FOR GLOBAL HEALTH INVOLVEMENT

7.8.1 Summary

Medical physics offers diverse career paths that significantly contribute to advancing global healthcare (Table 7.2). Through clinical practice, academia, research, industry, and global health initiatives, medical physicists address disparities in access to life-saving technologies while driving innovation and improving healthcare outcomes. Their collective efforts shape the future of healthcare and foster equitable solutions worldwide [18].

7.8.2 Opportunities for Global Health Involvement

7.8.2.1 Bridging the Global Health Gap

A defining feature of medical physics is its ability to reduce inequities in healthcare access, particularly in LMICs, where gaps in radiotherapy and diagnostic imaging persist. Medical physicists contribute by:

- **Expanding Infrastructure:** Collaborating with organizations like the IAEA, they establish radiotherapy centres, implement quality assurance protocols, and train local professionals.

- **Developing Sustainable Solutions:** Researchers and industry professionals create portable imaging systems and low-cost brachytherapy devices tailored for resource-limited settings.

TABLE 7.2 Comparison of the Five Major Career Paths in Medical Physics: Clinical Practice, Academia, Research, Industry, and Global Health Initiatives

Career Path	Primary Role	Key Responsibilities	Educational Requirements	Global Health Contributions
Clinical Practice	Provide patient-centred care through radiation safety, dosimetry, and equipment QA.	Dosimetry, quality assurance, equipment maintenance, and patient safety.	Master's or PhD + Residency + Certification (e.g., ABR, IMPCB).	Establish radiotherapy centres, train local staff, and ensure QA in LMICs.
Academia	Educate students and residents, conduct research, and shape academic programmes.	Teaching, mentoring, research, and leadership in academic programmes.	PhD in medical physics or related field + Research and teaching experience.	Develop curricula for underserved regions, build academic partnerships, and train local talent.
Research	Innovate and optimize medical technologies, focusing on diagnostic and therapeutic advancements.	Developing new technologies, radiation safety studies, and AI integration.	PhD + Postdoctoral training + Interdisciplinary collaboration skills.	Create affordable technologies, optimize treatment protocols, and advance AI applications.
Industry	Develop, test, and commercialize medical technologies; ensure regulatory compliance.	Product development, regulatory compliance, and technical support.	Master's or PhD + Regulatory Knowledge + Business acumen.	Design cost-effective solutions, transfer technology to underserved regions, and support sustainability.
Global health initiatives	Address healthcare disparities by improving access to cancer care and diagnostics in underserved regions.	Policy advocacy, capacity building, and infrastructure development.	Master's or PhD + Global health/Public health training + Cultural competence.	Expand access to care, advocate for policy changes, and strengthen local healthcare systems.

- **Building Local Capacity:** Academic physicists develop curricula and mentorship programmes to empower local professionals and ensure self-reliance.

These contributions collectively reduce the global cancer burden and improve health equity.

7.8.2.2 Driving Innovation

Innovation is central to medical physics, with professionals advancing technologies to enhance diagnosis and treatment:

- **Clinical Practice:** Optimizing treatment protocols and integrating technologies like adaptive radiotherapy to improve cancer care.

- **Academia:** Pioneering research in artificial intelligence, molecular imaging, and nanotechnology.

- **Industry:** Transforming research into practical, accessible solutions for global healthcare systems.

These advancements benefit both high-income countries and LMICs, ensuring that progress is inclusive and impactful.

7.8.2.3 Lifelong Learning and Collaboration

Medical physics demands continuous professional development to keep pace with evolving technologies. Certification programmes, workshops, and global conferences enable professionals to remain at the forefront of their field. Collaboration across disciplines – healthcare, engineering, data science, and policy-making – amplifies their impact, driving innovation, and holistic cancer care strategies.

7.8.2.4 The Future of Medical Physics

The profession's future lies in [19]:

- **Global Integration:** Strengthened collaborations between high-income countries and LMICs.

- **Emerging Technologies:** Innovations in AI, quantum imaging, and sustainability.

- **Equity and Access:** Expanding opportunities for underrepresented groups, ensuring diverse perspectives in global health initiatives.

Medical physicists play a transformative role in shaping global healthcare. By leveraging their expertise and embracing collaboration, they advance equity, innovation, and sustainability, making a lasting impact on healthcare systems worldwide.

REFERENCES

1. CAMPEP. Commission on Accreditation of Medical Physics Educational Programs (CAMPEP). [Accessed 2025-03-01]; Available from: http://www.campep.org/.

2. American Board of Radiology (ABR). [Accessed 2024-08-21]; Available from: https://www.theabr.org/.

3. International Medical Physics Certification Board (IMPCB). IMPCB. [Accessed: 2025-03-02]; Available from: https://www.impcbdb.org/about/.

4. Rosenblatt, E. and E. Zubizarreta, Radiotherapy in Cancer Care: Facing the Global Challenge. 2017, Vienna, Austria: International Atomic Energy Agency (IAEA) [Accessed 2025-03-02]; Available at https://www-pub.iaea.org/MTCD/Publications/PDF/P1638_web.pdf.

5. Grossi, R.M., The IAEA's Rays of Hope Leverages Nuclear Science and Collaboration to Fight Cancer in Developing Countries. *J Cancer Policy*, 2022. **34**: p. 100357.

6. Ngwa, W., *et al.*, Cancer in sub-Saharan Africa: A Lancet Oncology Commission. *Lancet Oncol*, 2022. **23**(6): p. e251–e312.

7. International Atomic Energy Agency (IAEA), Postgraduate Medical Physics Academic Programmes. TCS 56 (Rev.1). Training Course Series. 2021, Vienna, Austria: International Atomic Energy Agency.

8. Zubizarreta, E., J. Van Dyk, and Y. Lievens, Analysis of Global Radiotherapy Needs and Costs by Geographic Region and Income Level. *Clin Oncol (R Coll Radiol)*, 2017. **29**(2): p. 84–92.

9. Adewole, I.F., *et al.*, Brain Drain in Cancer Care: The Shrinking Clinical Oncology Workforce in Nigeria. *JCO Global Oncol*, 2023. **9**(1): p. e2300257.

10. Surbone, A., Cultural Aspects of Communication in Cancer Care, in *Communication in Cancer Care. Recent Results in Cancer Research*, F. Stiefel, Editor. 2006, Springer, Berlin, Heidelberg. p. 91–104.

11. Jaffray, D.A., *et al.*, Harnessing Progress in Radiotherapy for Global Cancer Control. *Nat. Cancer*, 2023. **4**: p. 1228–1238.

12. International Atomic Energy Agency (IAEA), Artificial Intelligence in Medical Physics. 2023, Vienna, Austria: International Atomic Energy Agency (IAEA) [Accessed 2025-03-02]; Available from: https://www.iaea.org/publications/15450/artificial-intelligence-in-medical-physics.

13. Chen, S., *et al.*, Estimates and Projections of the Global Economic Cost of 29 Cancers in 204 Countries and Territories From 2020 to 2050. *JAMA Oncol*, 2023. **9**(4): p. 465–472.

14. World Economic Forum, 6 Experts Reveal the Technologies Set to Revolutionize Cancer Care. 2024 [Accessed: 2025-03-02]; Available from: https://www.weforum.org/stories/2022/02/cancer-care-future-technology-experts/.

15. U.S. Food and Drug Administration (FDA). Premarket Notification 510(k). 2020 [Accessed: 2025-03-02]; Available from: https://www.fda.gov/medical-devices/premarket-submissions-selecting-and-preparing-correct-submission/premarket-notification-510k.

16. International Atomic Energy Agency (IAEA), *Radiotherapy Facilities: Master Planning and Concept Design Considerations*. IAEA Human Health Reports No. 10. 2014, Vienna, Austria: International Atomic Energy Agency (IAEA).
17. International Atomic Energy Agency (IAEA). *African Regional Cooperative Agreement for Research, Development and Training Related to Nuclear Science and Technology (AFRA) – Fifth Extension*. 2019 [Accessed: 2025-03-02]; Available from: https://www.iaea.org/sites/default/files/20/01/afra-brochure-2019.pdf.
18. Rehani, M.M., *et al.*, The International Organization for Medical Physics – A Driving Force for the Global Development of Medical Physics. Health Technol (Berl), 2022. **12**(3): p. 617–631.
19. Christofides, S., The Future of Medical Physics The Role of Medical Physics in Research and Development An Opinion, in *World Congress on Medical Physics and Biomedical Engineering*, September 7-12, 2009, O. Dössel and W.C. Schlegel, Editors. 2009, Springer Nature: Munich, Germany. p. 114–116.

CHAPTER 8

Mentoring in a Global Context

Kwan Hoong Ng and Jacob Van Dyk

8.1 CHAPTER OBJECTIVES

- To highlight the critical challenges faced by low- and middle-income countries (LMICs) in providing effective medical physics education and training

- To describe innovative methods for delivering medical physics education and training in resource-limited settings

- To explain the importance of various models of mentoring in medical physics

- To describe the key characteristics of mentoring support

- To explain the strategies and recommendations for developing effective mentoring programmes in medical physics

8.2 INTRODUCTION

As healthcare technology advances to improve both diagnosis and treatment, the demand rises for qualified medical physicists. However, the provision and standard of education and training vary greatly around the world, with a huge disparity between high-income countries (HICs) and low- and middle-income countries (LMICs). There is a definite need for robust and sustainable training programmes, particularly in LMICs. This chapter focuses on the global demand for mentorship in medical physics,

DOI: 10.1201/9781003527749-8

the challenges encountered, and methods to improve mentorship. The distribution of trained medical physicists is not balanced. HICs often have better training programmes and educational resources, while LMICs frequently deal with fewer educational options, a lack of qualified trainers, and weak infrastructure.

For the purpose of this chapter, we define the *mentor* to be a person with more experience or more knowledge in a specific area who helps guide and support the less experienced or less knowledgeable *mentee* in that specific area. Note that two equally knowledgeable and professionally experienced people could have a mentor/mentee relationship, for example concerning leadership or managerial skills [1].

8.3 NEEDS AND LIMITATIONS OF EDUCATION AND TRAINING IN LMICS

Expanding Demand: Worldwide, the demand for qualified and skilled medical physicists is growing fast to ensure optimum and safe use of sophisticated advanced technologies, such as those used in radiation therapy and diagnostic imaging (see Chapter 1 of this book). However, the number of trained medical physicists is insufficient to meet the demand, especially in LMICs.

Shortage of Formal Programmes: Many LMICs have very few or no formal medical physics education and training programmes. In cases where programmes exist, they often lack the proper infrastructure or resources to deliver good education. Consequently, early career medical physicists miss the foundational training needed to advance their clinical skills.

Lacking Training Tools: While in HICs, medical physicists are trained on the latest equipment and techniques, many LMICs lack modern training tools. The lack of resources, like linear accelerators or advanced imaging systems, hampers essential practical training.

Lack of Experienced Mentors: Another significant barrier to effective training in LMICs is the lack of experienced mentors. In such countries, medical physicists often work alone with few seniors to guide them, thus hampering their skill and career progression.

Lack of Financial Resources: Training programmes that involve hands-on experience with advanced technology are costly. Financial issues in LMICs make it difficult for institutions to invest in essential infrastructure, teaching tools, and qualified faculty.

8.4 METHODS OF PROVIDING EDUCATION AND TRAINING IN RESOURCE-LIMITED ENVIRONMENTS

Delivering education and training in medical physics in low-resource settings requires innovative strategies. Here we suggest a few methods that could help overcome such barriers and give aspiring medical physicists the chance to gain the necessary skills.

Virtual and Remote Learning: With increased internet access, virtual learning has become an effective way to provide education. Online courses, webinars, and virtual simulations could help convey important theoretical knowledge and practical skills, especially where physical training resources are limited. For instance, virtual reality (VR) and augmented reality (AR) could recreate clinical settings and procedures, serving as a budget-friendly alternative to hands-on training with actual equipment [2, 3].

Regional Training Centres and Partnerships: Cooperation between well-resourced institutions and those in LMICs could assist with education and training. Training centres could be set up as regional hubs for advanced learning. These centres would offer resources such as simulation tools, knowledgeable faculty, and networking opportunities with professionals from wealthier regions. Collaboration with global organizations, like the International Atomic Energy Agency (IAEA), could bring funding and technical assistance to help sustain these centres [4].

Mobile Training Programmes and Workshops: Mobile programmes, including workshops and seminars, could be put together to deliver education to regions with few formal schooling options [5]. These programmes could be temporary or semi-permanent and tailored to meet local needs. Expert trainers could travel to hospitals and medical schools to provide hands-on training in relevant medical physics techniques and equipment, particularly those suited to the local healthcare environment.

Learning via International Networks: Learning programmes connecting professionals in LMICs with experienced tutors in HICs are becoming more available. These online teaching–learning (mentoring) relationships enable learners (mentees) to gain expert advice, educational materials, and career guidance, regardless of where they are located. International networks, like the IAEA's virtual university

[6] for the medical physics community, offer online courses and a broad expert panel. Medical Physics for World Benefit (MPWB) [7] has developed the *Open Syllabus* project [8]. This project connects freely accessible online materials directly with the syllabus components of the IAEA TC-37 report [9] on training requirements for medical physics residents specializing in radiation oncology. Other specialties are being considered for the future.

8.5 MENTORING MODELS IN MEDICAL CONNECTING PROFESSIONALS

Various mentoring models have been developed and evolved based on available resources, intended training levels, and programme objectives.

Formal Mentoring: This programme typically includes a structured curriculum and matches mentors and mentees according to specific career or educational objectives. They suit institutions with resources for training and progress evaluation.

Group Mentoring: This model permits several mentees to gain from one or more mentors, encourages collaboration among mentees, and is especially useful in settings where mentor availability is low.

Informal Peer Mentorship: Peer mentoring allows mentees at similar career stages to support one another, akin to the "buddy system." This is particularly useful in situations where fewer senior mentors are available. Peer mentors share knowledge, work together on problem solving, and provide advice based on their experiences.

Table 8.1 compares various mentoring types and gives some of the pros and cons of each.

8.6 BASICS OF MENTORING SUPPORT

Customized Mentoring: Mentoring should be customized to meet the unique needs based on mentees' situation, career stage, and goals, and mentoring should be customized to meet these varied needs. For instance, a new graduate may require more frequent support to build confidence in clinical experience, while a more advanced mentee might need specific advice on advanced technologies or starting a research project.

TABLE 8.1   Types of Mentoring and Their Pros and Cons

Mentoring Type	Description	Pros	Cons
One-on-one, face-to-face (informal)	Mentoring that occurs spontaneously or at an individual's request. May have a specific purpose or it may be more general without specific goals being defined.	Avoids requirements of structured programme. May aid the development of personal relationships.	The lack of structure means that no specific goals are defined in that there are no metrics for defining success, or when to terminate the mentorship.
One-on-one, face-to-face (formal)	Formal mentorship means that specific goals are defined, reviews of the success of mentorship are carried out, and when to terminate the mentorship is defined.	With specific objectives, metrics, and reviews, the likelihood of success increases.	Involves more bureaucracy which may or may not impede progress.
One-on-one, virtual (formal or informal)	Remote mentorship using information and communications technologies (ICTs). Could be formal through an organization, or informal through personal contacts.	Allows mentorship when mentors may not be available locally.	Direct face-to-face interaction will not be possible. This is especially relevant for medical physicists when they are dealing with hands-on experiences either with dosimetry procedures or dealing with patient-related procedures.
Group mentoring	Could involve one mentor with several mentees. Or it could involve several mentors with several mentees. The group meets regularly to discuss various topics.	The peer group under the guidance of the mentor helps develop each other's skills and knowledge. Provides perspectives from different experiences.	It's difficult to develop confidence and relationships with individuals. Because of multiple attendees, it is more difficult to address individual questions.

Motivational Mentoring: Besides offering advice, a mentor should also care about the mentee's general well-being. Mentors need to meet regularly with mentees, whether in person or online, providing useful feedback and acknowledging accomplishments. Consistent support is crucial as it keeps mentees motivated and focused on achieving their goals.

Context-Sensitive Mentoring: Mentors need to appreciate equity, diversity, and inclusivity (EDI) in cultural, social, and local realities. In some countries, mentoring is influenced by customs, and methods effective in one place may not work in another. Knowing the local cultural context is crucial for establishing trust and connections between mentors and mentees.

Mentoring by Accompaniment: Mentoring is a journey that goes on for a long time. Effective mentoring programmes focus on building lasting relationships that provide help at different stages of the mentee's career. Mentors need to keep communicating regularly, helping mentees with their career growth and career decisions.

Figure 8.1 summarizes some of the roles associated with mentoring.

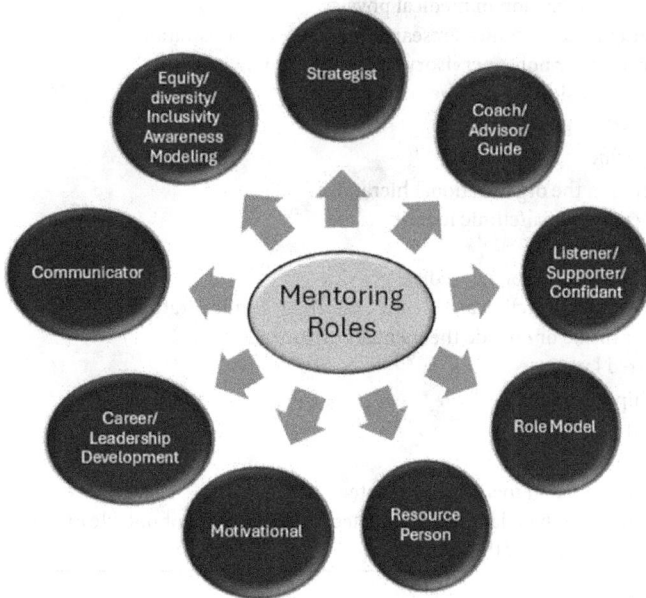

FIGURE 8.1   A summary of some of the key roles that can be addressed in the mentoring process.

8.7 MATCHING MENTOR AND MENTEE

Mentoring should be customized to meet the unique needs based on the mentees' situation, career stage, and goals. For instance, a new graduate may require more frequent support to build confidence in clinical experience, while a more advanced mentee might need specific advice on advanced technologies or starting a research project. Table 8.2 summarizes some of the considerations for matching mentor and mentee.

8.8 DEVELOPING EFFICIENT MENTORING PROGRAMMES

Creating and implementing successful mentoring programmes require a critical understanding of the mentoring process, a willingness to collaborate, and strategic planning. The following approaches are recommended:

TABLE 8.2 Information to Be Obtained by Mentors and Mentees Regarding Primary Mentoring Relationships

Mentor specific
- Location in the organizational hierarchy
- Gender and racial/ethnic identity
- Career stage
- Career specialization in medical physics
- Career emphasis (clinical, research teaching, administration)
- Supervisory or nonsupervisory relationship to mentee
- Inside or outside the mentee's organization
- Preferred language

Mentee specific
- Location in the organizational hierarchy
- Gender and racial/ethnic identity
- Career stage
- Career specialization in medical physics
- Career emphasis (clinical, research, teaching, administration)
- Mentor inside or outside the mentee's organization
- Preferred language

Relationship specific
- Formal or informal
- Relationship duration
- Age differential of mentor and mentee
- Who initiated the relationship (mentee, mentor, inside or outside organization)
- Closeness/quality of the relationship

Source: Adapted from [10].

Creating a Framework: Professional organizations, such as MPWB, could develop a standardized mentoring framework to ensure that mentorship programmes are well structured and effective. This framework should include guidelines for programme duration, how mentors and mentees are matched, and parameters for successful implementation.

Utilizing Digital Technology: Digital tools should be maximized for online classes, webinars, video calls, and virtual simulations to enhance global mentoring. Additionally, fostering international collaboration could bridge the gap between HICs and LMICs.

Regular Assessment and Review: Mentorship programmes should be regularly reviewed and assessed to determine their effectiveness. By collecting feedback from both mentors and mentees, programmes could be refined and optimized. Criteria for assessment should include career growth, skill acquisition, and the broader impact of mentoring on healthcare results.

8.9 GLOBAL LEADERSHIP VIA MENTORING PROGRAMME

The Medical Physics Leadership and Mentoring Programme (MPLMP) was initiated in 2016 [11, 12].

Objectives: The MPLMP aims to develop leadership roles among young medical physicists, and to provide them with guidance and support. The programme, which began with 12 mentees, has since expanded to more than 30 members from regions including Asia, Latin America, and Africa. MPLMP seeks to foster professional growth and cultivate leadership skills through mentorship, inspired by Professor Ng's own experiences as a mentee to the late Professor John Cameron.

Approaches: This mentoring initiative combines traditional and e-mentoring (or virtual mentoring) approaches, allowing for communication between mentors and mentees from various parts of the world. The use of digital tools, like WhatsApp, Zoom, and Google Classroom, facilitates regular interactions and project collaborations, transcending geographic and time-zone barriers. Online mentoring sessions are held regularly, where mentees engage with mentors, share experiences, and discuss leadership development.

Access: MPLMP has created a global network of medical physicists, offering mentees access to experienced professionals and leaders in medical physics. The initiative has encouraged scientific collaboration, resulting in peer-reviewed publications and conference presentations. Additionally, MPLMP has used social media and websites to disseminate information about its activities and to promote gender equity within its membership.

Skills Enhancement: A survey of mentees showed that they have enhanced their leadership skills and widened their horizons in their professional roles. Most mentees reported improvements in skills, such as organization, technical aspects of their work, and writing of papers. Mentors also gained benefits from MPLMP, in which interactions with mentees were stimulating and rewarding.

Leadership: Challenges include coordination across various time zones and cultural backgrounds, but the programme has demonstrated resilience through the use of virtual mentoring. Looking ahead, MPLMP plans to expand by recruiting more mentees from Africa and Europe and engaging more mentors. The goal is to create a global network that promotes leadership in medical physics, ensuring that more professionals are prepared for future leadership roles in the healthcare industry.

Positive Outcomes: Based on its progress over the last eight years, MPLMP has made significant strides in developing the next generation of leaders in medical physics. Its global, collaborative model has shown positive outcomes for both mentees and mentors, with plans for further expansion and improvement to enhance its reach and effectiveness.

8.10 VIRTUAL MENTORING

8.10.1 Virtual Mentoring

Ideally, mentoring is undertaken in real time, face-to-face, and with local mentors in the work environment or even from nearby clinics or universities. However, as described above for the MPLMP programme, local mentors might not always be available because the expertise for the purpose of mentoring is lacking, or, as in lower-income contexts, there might be very few medical physics experts available to support a mentoring process.

In such cases, virtual mentoring using information and communications technologies (ICTs) would become the mentoring alternative.

8.10.2 Medical Physics for World Benefit (MPWB) Global Survey

Medical Physics for World Benefit (MPWB) undertook an online global perceptions survey to provide guidance on best approaches for virtual mentoring [1]. The survey links were sent to various known national, international, and regional medical physics organizations, as well as the Global MedPhys listserv, with these contacts possibly representing 30,000 medical physicists. There were nearly 400 responders from 76 countries with one-third representing LMICs. Sixty-eight percent were male and 32% female. The LMIC responders were generally younger with less working experience compared to the HIC responders. Fifty percent had an MSc and 44% with PhD. Fifty-eight percent specialized in radiation oncology medical physics, 25% in diagnostic imaging, and 16% in health physics with a number of individuals having multiple specializations. Thirty-eight percent had a lot of mentoring experience and 23% with a lot of mentee experience. Fifteen percent were interested in virtual mentoring as a mentee, 32% as a mentor, and 36% as both. The survey provided suggestions for guidance in setting up a virtual mentorship programme. These are summarized in the recommendation section below.

8.11 SUMMARY AND RECOMMENDATIONS

8.11.1 Summary

Bridging the Gap: Mentoring plays a critical role in addressing the global disparity in medical physics education and training. While HICs have access to advanced resources, LMICs face significant challenges, including limited infrastructure and few qualified mentors. By utilizing innovative approaches like virtual learning, regional centres, and mobile workshops, the gap could be bridged. The Medical Physics Leadership and Mentoring Programme exemplifies the positive impact of international collaboration. Mentoring, whether face-to-face or virtual, provides valuable support and development opportunities, fosters leadership, and ensures the growth of a skilled global medical physics workforce to meet increasing healthcare demands.

Appropriate Approaches: Effective mentoring is crucial to the development of medical physicists worldwide, especially in underserved regions. By adopting thoughtful, culturally sensitive, and technology-enabled approaches to mentoring, we could ensure that medical physicists receive the support and guidance they need to advance in their careers. By fostering international collaborations, standardizing mentorship frameworks, and committing to long-term sustainability, we could create successful global medical physics mentoring programmes that would have a lasting impact on healthcare systems worldwide.

8.11.2 Recommendations

1. Mentoring for medical physicists is an important component of professional development. Every medical physicist should seek mentors throughout their careers to address various aspects of career and knowledge development, be they related to technical skills, research guidance, leadership development, or simply improvement in daily functionality.

2. In recognition of inequities in mentoring resources around the globe, virtual mentoring may be the option of choice, especially for those working in a resource-constrained environment.

3. The MPWB mentoring survey suggests the following for the development of a structured mentoring process [1]:

    a) Obtain applications from potential mentors and mentees Including details on technical expertise, technologies in use, job role, and expectations.

    b) Match mentor and mentee through personal connections, local healthcare facility or university, professional/regional medical physics associations or MPWB.

    c) Note that while personal connections appear to be the preferred option for many, especially those in lower-income contexts, where there are fewer medical physicists, such connections may not be readily available; hence, a link to an organization may be more amenable.

    d) Provide appropriate training for mentor and mentee [13, 14].

    e) Mentor and mentee should jointly document a formal mentorship agreement. There are multiple sample agreements available on the internet. An example from the University of Alberta can be found here [15].

        i. Define expectations.

        ii. Define expected frequency, length, and format of meetings.

        iii. Define review process.

        iv. Timing and frequency of reviews.

    v. Assess successes and shortcomings.

    vi. Define length of time of mentorship commitment.

    vii. Include criteria for continuation or termination.

  f) Review total mentorship programme on a mutually established regular basis (possibly annually) and make amendments as needed. Example metrics for review can be found in the literature [13].

REFERENCES

1. Van Dyk, J., *et al.*, Virtual Mentoring for Medical Physicists: Results of a Global Online Survey. *J Med Phys*, 2024. **49**: p. 687–700.
2. Lastrucci, A., *et al.*, The Application of Virtual Environment Radiotherapy for RTT Training: A Scoping Review. *J Med Imaging Radiat Sci*, 2024. **55**(2): p. 339–346.
3. Chamunyonga, C., *et al.*, Utilising the Virtual Environment for Radiotherapy Training System to Support Undergraduate Teaching of IMRT, VMAT, DCAT Treatment Planning, and QA Concepts. *J Med Imaging Radiat Sci*, 2018. **49**(1): p. 31–38.
4. Grossi, R.M., The IAEA's Rays of Hope Leverages Nuclear Science and Collaboration to Fight Cancer in Developing Countries. *J Cancer Policy*, 2022. **34**: p. 100357.
5. Klimova, B., Mobile Learning in Medical Education. *J Med Syst*, 2018. **42**(10): p. 194.
6. International Atomic Energy Agency (IAEA). Human Health Campus. [Accessed 2024-08-21]; Available from: https://www.iaea.org/resources/databases/human-health-campus.
7. Medical Physics for World Benefit. [Accessed 2024-08-21]; Available from: www.mpwb.org.
8. Medical Physics for World Benefit (MPWB). Open Syllabus Project. 2024 [Accessed 2024-12-30]; Available from: https://mpwb.org/resources/Documents/OpenSyllabus/output.html.
9. International Atomic Energy Agency (IAEA), *Clinical Training of Medical Physicists Specializing in Radiation Oncology. TCS 37.* 2009, Vienna, Austria: International Atomic Energy Agency (IAEA).
10. Haggard, D.L., *et al.*, Who Is a Mentor? A Review of Evolving Definitions and Implications for Research. *J Manage*, 2011. **37**(1): p. 280–304.
11. Ng, A.H., Sirico, A.C.A., Lopez, A.H., Hoang, A.T., Chi, D.D., Prasetio, H., Uwadiae, I.B., Santos, J.C., Chhoert, K., Thomas, L.A., Giansante, L., Goulart, L., Rojas, L.J., Lubis, L.E., Yeh, M.Y., Pham, N.T., Trejo-Garcia, P.M., Cheng, S.C.S., Dang Quoc, S., Danghangthum, T., Ath, V., Guerra, V.H., Lin, Y.H., Bezak, E., Jeraj, R., Kron, T., Ng, K.H., Nurturing a Global Initiative in Medical Physics Leadership and Mentoring. *Med Phys Int*, 2020. **8**(3): p. 467–474.

12. Santos, J.C., *et al.*, Leadership and Mentoring in Medical Physics: The Experience of a Medical Physics International Mentoring Program. *Phys Med*, 2020. **76**: p. 337–344.
13. Chi, B.H., *et al.*, Evaluating Academic Mentorship Programs in Low- and Middle-Income Country Institutions: Proposed Framework and Metrics. *Am J Trop Med Hyg*, 2019. **100**(1_Suppl): p. 36–41.
14. Gandhi, M., *et al.*, Mentoring the Mentors: Implementation and Evaluation of Four Fogarty-Sponsored Mentoring Training Workshops in Low-and Middle-Income Countries. *Am J Trop Med Hyg*, 2019. **100**(1_Suppl): p. 20–28.
15. University of Alberta. Mentor and Mentee Orientations. 2023 [Accessed 2023-06-28]; Available from: https://albertamentorship.ca/resources/mentor-mentee-orientations/.

CHAPTER 9

Global Collaboration: Successes and Barriers

Jacob Van Dyk, Mauro Carrara,
Egor Titovich, and May Abdel-Wahab

9.1 CHAPTER OBJECTIVES

- To describe how we can learn from successes and failures in global collaborations
- To discuss barriers to global collaborations
  - Political, logistical, cultural
- To provide examples of how successes can be developed
- To consider factors that help overcome barriers to global collaboration
- To provide recommendations on developing successful global medical physics collaborations.

9.2 INTRODUCTION

Collaboration among stakeholders at regional and global levels is often advocated as a means of improving healthcare developments, effectively and efficiently, especially in low- to middle-income countries (LMICs) [1]. The question is: "Do these collaborations always work?" If not, what lessons can we learn from successes and failures of such collaborations to avoid issues that have fostered failures and to enhance the probability of

DOI: 10.1201/9781003527749-9

success? To answer this question, we first need to define what is a "success" and what is a "failure"?

Global collaboration was already defined in Chapter 1 as the act or process of voluntarily working together, generally involving efforts among individuals, institutions, or organizations from different geographical locations to share knowledge, resources, and insights for collective learning and progress [2]. "Success" in the context of global collaboration is defined as achieving the goal set out by the collaboration [3]. In contrast, "failure" occurs when a defined goal is not achieved, or it has been achieved in the short run but has not been sustained in the long run.

9.3 WHAT MAKES A GLOBAL HEALTHCARE PARTNERSHIP SUCCESSFUL?

Successful collaboration in healthcare teams can be attributed to numerous factors including interpersonal relationships within the team (interactional determinants), conditions within the organization (organizational determinants), and the organization's environment (systemic determinants) [4]. In their review of the literature, San Martin-Rodriguez *et al.* [4] found that collaboration within a team requires the presence of a series of elements in the relationships between team members. These include a willingness to collaborate, trust in each other, mutual respect, and communication. Furthermore, organizational determinants also play a crucial role, especially in terms of human resource management and strong leadership.

The systematic literature review by Guilfoyle *et al.* [3] found 26 articles that described healthcare partnerships between high- and low-income countries, which involved a primary goal revolving around medical education, training, and curriculum development. Only two of the partnerships had achieved a self-sustaining programme over ten years. Lack of funding was identified as a major barrier to sustainability. The following guidelines were proposed to improve the chances of a successful and sustainable collaboration:

1. The partnership should be initiated by the host country or through joint decision between partners. The partnership goals, expectations, and responsibilities should be clearly outlined.

2. A needs assessment should be performed prior to embarking on any project. All stakeholders should be involved in this needs assessment.

3. Stakeholders should engage the Ministry of Health or local government during their needs assessment and project planning.

4. A comprehensive ten-year fiscal budget should be devised, avoiding heavy reliance on charitable and private donations, and considering opportunities for income-generating activities.

5. The project should be specifically tailored to match local need, cultural practices, local infrastructure, and operative budget.

6. The project should, at minimum, have a five- to ten-year plan which incorporates a graduated shift of responsibility to the host partner and a clear exit strategy of the visiting partner, with the caveat that continued financial support from the visiting partner even though human resources and expertise are no longer required.

9.4 DATA GENERATION FOR INFORMING SUCCESSFUL COLLABORATIONS

To attain data for guiding policy-makers and enhancing evidence-based decision-making, a collaboration on the development of databases and data collection is essential. Examples here include the development of the International Atomic Energy (IAEA) databases such as Directory of Radiotherapy Centres (DIRAC) [5], the Directory of Nuclear Medicine Centers (NUMDAB) [6], and the IAEA Medical Imaging and Nuclear Medicine Global Database (IMAGINE) [7], all of which have supported Lancet Oncology Commissions [8–10]. On a wider scale, an analysis based on the use of DIRAC as a resource for publications on health economics topics can also help identify trends in healthcare partnerships between high-income countries (HICs) and LMICs. Publications referring to DIRAC in the time frame between 2012 and 2023 were considered. Among the 253 peer-reviewed publications identified, 176 publications dealing with health economics topics were scrutinized. The year of publication, the number of authors, and the income of the country of their affiliation were analyzed. The results show that there has been a steady increase in publications dealing with health economics topics referring to DIRAC since 2012 (Figure 9.1a). Out of the selected 176 publications, 69 (39%) and 25 (14%) were drafted by authors affiliated only to institutions in HICs and LMICs, respectively. The remaining 82 (47%) are the result of partnerships between researchers belonging to both HICs and LMICs.

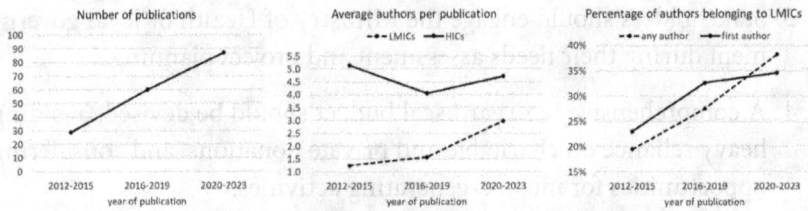

FIGURE 9.1 (a) Number of publications dealing with health economics topics referring to DIRAC data published between 2012 and 2023; (b) average number of authors per publication belonging to institutions in LMICs (dotted line) and HICs (solid line); (c) percentage of authors (dotted line), and first authors only (solid line), belonging to institutions in LMICs, compared to the overall number of authors.

The significant increase in the number of authors belonging to institutions in LMICs – from 149 (2012–2015), to 243 (2016–2019), to 410 (2020–2023) – contributed to the rise in the average number of authors per publication affiliated with institutions in LMICs (Figure 9.1b). A similar trend was not observed for the average number of authors per publication affiliated with institutions in HICs, as the highest figure was recorded during the first four-year period (2012–2015). The percentage of authors belonging to institutions in LMICs, compared to the overall number of authors contributing to the analyzed publications, almost doubled over the studied time. The increase in the percentage of authors from institutions in LMICs serving as first authors has slowed down over the last four years (Figure 9.1c). The geographical distribution of authors' affiliations (as of the end of 2021) is given in Figure 9.2.

Several findings can be deduced from this analysis, which may help interpret trends and challenges in global healthcare partnerships:

1. Access to global data fosters collaboration among research teams worldwide. International organizations, such as the IAEA, play a key role in this effort by providing open-source resources (e.g., databases) that serve as fundamental support for researchers globally.

2. There are several instances of partnerships among researchers belonging to developed and developing countries in the field of health economics linked to radiotherapy, showcasing virtuous examples.

3. Publications authored by researchers from LMICs are more often the result of collaborations with researchers belonging to developed countries than the opposite.

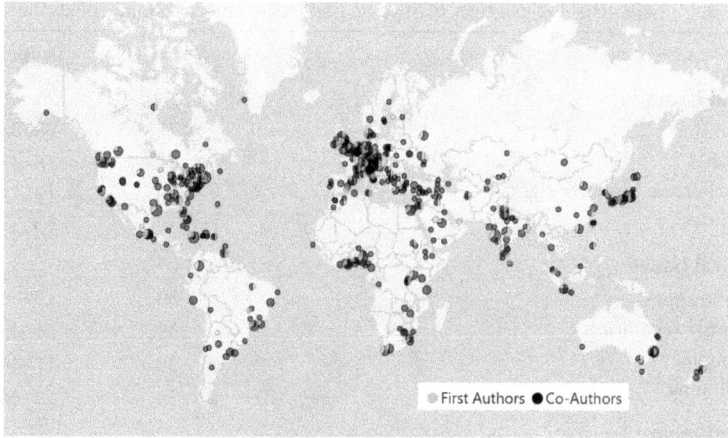

FIGURE 9.2   Geographical distribution of authors' affiliations of papers dealing with health economics topics referring to DIRAC data.

4. The number of authors from institutions in LMICs, as well as their representation per publication, is increasing significantly, indicating greater involvement of institutions from LMICs.

5. Leadership by researchers from developing countries in conducting health economics studies and drafting publications should be encouraged and supported to further strengthen sustainable research capacity in LMICs.

9.5 BARRIERS TO GLOBAL COLLABORATION

In a study gauging scientists' attitudes and experiences with international collaborations, over 9,400 biologists and physicists from eight countries/regions – the United States, the United Kingdom, India, Italy, Taiwan, Hong Kong, Turkey, and France – were surveyed [11]. While most scientists claimed international collaboration was important, their actual participation in such collaborations was much lower. They identified the rates of three types of barriers – political, logistical, and cultural – based on categories developed in previous studies. Moreover, they identified nine additional categories of barriers including lack of funding for international work, restrictions on material and data sharing, and differences in academic standards. Table 9.1 summarizes these scientists' perspectives on specific barriers to international collaboration. Respondents also complained about bias against scholars from lower-income countries. Their study highlights areas where efforts could be made to address policy

TABLE 9.1 Scientists' Perspectives of Specific Barriers to International Collaboration

	Mean (%)	Range (%)
Political Issues		
• Funding	77	68–85
• Visas	31	18–43
• Intellectual property rights	20	13–25
• Politics	7	5.3–11
Logistical Issues		
• Time zones	30	13–55
• Family separation	39	31–45
• Language	35	17–49
• Calendar	39	22–36
Cultural Issues		
• Ethics	18	15–20
• Gender	6	0.0–11
• Religion	3	1.2–4.7
• Sexual orientation	1	0.4–2.4

Note: The percent of "yes" responses to each barrier surveyed is shown, as values averaged over the eight countries/regions. The range between minimum and maximum values is also shown.
Source: Adapted from [11].

issues, institutional barriers, and national biases to promote more productive collaboration in the global scientific community.

Note that this specific paper addresses the responses from biologists and physicists from these specific countries/regions. While the results provide a representative sampling for basic scientists, it is likely that if medical physicists were surveyed, some of the results might show similar trends. In another review [12], the authors examined the existing literature of collaboration to determine a set of factors foundational to a framework of collaboration failure. However, as a starting point, they looked at the factors that made the collaboration a success (Table 9.2).

A further analysis looked at topics that could be linked to collaborative failure. They looked at three different categorization types: (1) agency-based, which includes members from public institutions such as government agencies, universities, or other interest groups, (2) citizen-based, which is primarily composed of private citizens that work to address community level issues, and (3) mixed collaborations, which are somewhere between citizen-based and agency-based. The results are shown in Table 9.3 and are categorized into three themes: organizational dynamics, interorganizational processes, and management.

TABLE 9.2   Condensed List of Collaboration "Success" factors

- Everybody brings assets to the table/shared resources/information
- Common goals/shared vision
- Assumption of shared risk
- Voluntary participation
- Mutual benefit/resource allocation
- Interdependence
- Flat, not hierarchical, organization/consensus decision-making/design
- Social capital/trust/communication
- Diverse stakeholders/leadership/key personnel
- Formality of the agreement
- Organizational autonomy/resolution of turf issues

Source: Adapted from [12].

TABLE 9.3   Relative Importance of Factor Impacting Collaboration Failure

	Collaboration Type	
Factor	Agency-Based	Citizen-Based
Success (Process or Output)	O	P
Organizational Dynamics		
Value differences	L	H
Divergent goals	H	H
Resource constraints	H	M
Time constraints	M	H
Stakeholder involvement	M	H
Staff support	H	L
Interorganizational Processes		
Power imbalance	H	L
Established rules/documentation	H	L
Conflict resolution	M	H
Role definition	H	H
Communications	M	H
Planning	H	H
Need for interdependence	H	L
Government structures	H	L
Management		
Trust, legitimacy, social capital	L	H
Skilled convener	M	H
Managing perspectives	M	H
Environmental/local constraints	L	H

Note: L = low, M = medium, H = high.
Source: Adapted from [12].

These results provide a framework of consideration when addressing collaborations, whether agency-based or citizen-based, and can be used as a barometer to review the collaboration with a corresponding importance level regarding specific failure factors.

At a public health level, Woldetsadik *et al.* [13] performed a qualitative evaluation of enabling factors and barriers to the success and sustainability of national public health institutes (NPHIs) in Cambodia, Colombia, Liberia, Mozambique, Nigeria, Rwanda, and Zambia by performing semi-structured, in-person interviews. Participants identified five enabling factors critical to the success and sustainability of NPHIs: (1) strong leadership, (2) financial autonomy, (3) political commitment and country ownership, (4) strengthening capacity of NPHI staff, and (5) forming strategic partnerships. Three themes emerged related to major barriers or threats to the sustainability of NPHIs: (1) reliance on partner funding to maintain key activities, (2) changes in NPHI leadership, and (3) staff attrition and turnover. This study informs country leadership on how to direct efforts to strengthen and sustain NPHIs and also provides considerations for other types of collaborative efforts.

9.6 EXAMPLE CASE HISTORY

9.6.1 Sustainability of Radiotherapy Services

Chapter 6 of this book addresses factors that contribute to a sustainable health-related programme. The chapter included a table (Figure 6.4) of data showing the number of radiotherapy machines in 34 different countries in Africa by year since 1991. Some of these countries lacked continuous sustainable use of these machines.

The development and sustainability of a radiotherapy programme depend on several key factors: a well-educated and trained workforce, commitment and support from decision-makers alongside local political stability, and properly maintained equipment and facility infrastructure. If any of these components fails, the long-term viability of the programme is at risk [14] and might result in a decline of services over time. The following expands on these potential barriers.

1. **Well-Educated and Trained Workforce:** In countries where there is a lack of experienced professionals to provide local education and clinical training, international support becomes essential for staff training and continuous professional development. This reliance

significantly increases the costs and challenges of developing a sustainable radiotherapy programme. Additionally, brain drain is a concern in many cases. When services are not functioning effectively or when staff roles, responsibilities, and professional recognition (e.g., the acknowledgement of clinically qualified medical physicists as healthcare professionals) are inadequate, professionals are more likely to migrate to countries with higher living standards and better working conditions.

2. **Commitment and Support from Decision-Makers Alongside Local Political Stability:** While international organizations and institutions may offer significant support, local commitment from decision-makers is a critical cornerstone for a sustainable programme. Political instability has frequently been shown to disrupt the continuity of services. Furthermore, the establishment and enforcement of adequate legal and regulatory radiation protection frameworks are essential for the programme's success.

3. **Properly Maintained Equipment and Facility Infrastructure:** Equipment must be preserved and maintained to ensure reliable operation. Preventive and corrective maintenance over the entire lifetime for major equipment and information technology systems, including the availability of spare parts when required, should be established and accessible. Additionally, stable electricity, access to clean water, and effective climate control systems for regulating temperature and humidity are vital for the uninterrupted operation of radiotherapy equipment and the uptime of radiotherapy treatment machines.

When designing new projects, these factors should be thoroughly addressed and carefully planned to enhance the likelihood that newly established or expanded radiotherapy programmes will be safe, sustainable, and effective.

9.6.2 The IAEA Rays of Hope Anchor Centres

The IAEA Rays of Hope Anchor Centres [15–17] are specialized institutions designated by the IAEA to function as key hubs for training, capacity-building, quality assurance, and research innovation in radiation medicine (i.e., radiation oncology, nuclear medicine, diagnostic radiology, and medical physics).

These centres are recognized as regional leaders, contributing to best practices in radiation medicine and support continuing professional development through integrated cancer services with a range of modern technologies. Anchor Centres have demonstrated resilience and long-lasting experience working with the IAEA to support their respective regions. They have a proven track record of collaboration and joint activities in several areas, including:

- Participation in coordinated research projects
- Training of fellows (generally additional training for up to one year)
- Support for IAEA training courses and missions
- Provision of education and training programmes in radiation medicine-related disciplines.

The IAEA Global Anchor Centres network presents a unique opportunity for worldwide collaboration aimed at continuous improvement of cancer management across all world regions. Moreover, it fosters South–South Cooperation, as many Anchor Centres are located in developing countries. These centres will continue to support their regions, with the IAEA intending to provide them support to further enhance their educational and research capacities and infrastructures. By joining this IAEA global network, Anchor Centres will optimize and pool resources, establish direct communication channels, and develop integrated procedures and protocols.

9.7 SUMMARY AND RECOMMENDATIONS

9.7.1 Summary

Collaboration among stakeholders at regional and global levels provides a means of improving healthcare developments, especially in LMICs. The characteristics of successful collaboration include willingness to collaborate, mutual trust, respect, and communication. Organizational determinants also play a crucial role, especially in terms of human resource management and strong leadership. Broad guidelines for successful partnerships include project initiation by host country, performing a needs assessment prior to developing the project, engaging the relevant stakeholders during the needs assessment and project planning, development of a long-term budget, tailoring project to match local circumstances along with a five- to ten-year plan with a clear transfer of responsibility and ownership to the host organization or country. Availability of appropriate data will help guide policy-makers and enhance evidence-based decision-making. Examples of databases developed at the IAEA that provide guidance data are provided. The IAEA's Rays of Hope initiative is a model of how South–South cooperation can be encouraged to develop radiotherapy capacity in LMICs.

9.7.2 Recommendations

The following are recommendations aimed at increasing the probability of success of development programmes or even smaller projects. They are based on the experiences as published in the peer-reviewed literature. While trying to be generic, these recommendations likely need to be adapted according to the nature of the project, the partners involved, and the local circumstances.

1. Ideally, partnerships for larger programmes or smaller projects would be initiated by the host organization or country, thus demonstrating a strong interest and ownership of the development activity. At times, these could be generated through meetings with the mutual involvement of the development organization and the host.

2. With the involvement of all stakeholders, a needs assessment should be performed prior to embarking on any project. The needs assessment should be data driven and make appropriate use of relevant databases according to the subject at hand.

3. Metrics should be developed at the beginning of the project to determine its success and should be reviewed on a regular basis to evaluate needs for adaptation should modifications be required.

4. As part of the project planning process, stakeholders should engage the appropriate authoritative bodies such as the Ministry of Health, or local government, or local university during their needs assessment and project planning stages.

5. Be aware of potential project barriers as they might relate to power imbalances between donor and host partners in priority-setting and decision-making. Potential equity issues relate to asymmetries of voice and participation and the development of criteria related

to evaluation. Decisions are often biased by the voices from HICs, despite programmes being developed for LMICs.

6. To develop sustainability in the long run, a comprehensive long-term (e.g., ten-year) fiscal budget should be devised, avoiding heavy reliance on charitable and private donations, and considering opportunities for income-generating activities.

7. The project should be specifically tailored to match local need, cultural practices, local infrastructure, and the corresponding operative budget.

8. The project should, at minimum, have a five- to ten-year plan which incorporates a graduated shift of responsibility to the host partner and a clear exit strategy of the visiting partner, with the caveat of continued agreed-upon financial support from the visiting partner even though their human resources and expertise are no longer required.

9. Organizers of larger programmes and smaller projects should be aware of potential barriers to the success of development projects based on the broad topics of political, logistical, and cultural issues (Table 9.1) and organizational dynamics, interorganizational processes, and management (Table 9.3).

10. Open communication with all the stakeholders throughout the entire project will enhance its likelihood of success. Regular progress reports describing both successes and failures allow for encouragement of continuity as well as adaptation as needed. More formal reports published in the peer-reviewed literature will provide outcome benefits for others involved in similar projects.

REFERENCES

1. Abdel-Wahab, M., *et al.*, Global Radiotherapy: Current Status and Future Directions-White Paper. *JCO Glob Oncol*, 2021. **7**: p. 827–842.
2. Castaner, X. and N. Oliveira, Collaboration, Coordination, and Cooperation Among Organizations: Establishing the Distinctive Meanings of These Terms through a Systematic Literature Review. *J Manage*, 2020. **46**(6): p. 965–1001.
3. Guilfoyle, R., A.D. Morzycki, and A. Saleh, What Makes Global Healthcare Partnerships Successful? A Systematic Review. *Glob Public Health*, 2022. **17**(5): p. 662–671.

4. San Martin-Rodriguez, L., *et al.*, The Determinants of Successful Collaboration: A Review of Theoretical And Empirical Studies. *J Interprof Care*, 2005. **19 Suppl 1**: p. 132–47.

5. International Atomic Energy Agency (IAEA). Directory of Radiotherapy Centres, DIRAC. [Accessed 2025-01-16]; Available from: https://dirac.iaea.org/.

6. International Atomic Energy Agency (IAEA). Nuclear Medicine Centers, NUMDAB. [Accessed 2025-01-16]; Available from: https://nucmedicine.iaea.org/statistics/infrastructure.

7. International Atomic Energy Agency (IAEA). IAEA Medical Imaging and Nuclear Medicine Global Resources Database, IMAGINE. [Accessed 2025-01-16]; Available from: https://humanhealth.iaea.org/HHW/DBStatistics/IMAGINE.html.

8. Hricak, H., et al., Medical Imaging and nuclear Medicine: A Lancet Oncology Commission. *Lancet Oncol*, 2021. **22**(4): p. e136–e172.

9. Abdel-Wahab, M., *et al.*, Radiotherapy and Theranostics: a Lancet Oncology Commission. *Lancet Oncol*, 2024. **25**(11): p. e545–e580.

10. Atun, R., et al., Expanding Global Access to Radiotherapy. *Lancet Oncol*, 2015. **16**(10): p. 1153–1186.

11. Matthews, K.R.W., *et al.*, International Scientific Collaborative Activities and Barriers to Them in Eight Societies. *Account Res*, 2020. **27**(8): p. 477–495.

12. McNamara, M.W., K. Miller-Stevens, and J.C. Morris, Exploring Determinants of Collaboration Failure. *Int J Public Admin*, 2020. **43**(1): p. 49–59.

13. Woldetsadik, M.A., *et al.*, Qualitative Evaluation Of Enabling Factors and Barriers to the Success and Sustainability of National Public Health Institutes in Cambodia, Colombia, Liberia, Mozambique, Nigeria, Rwanda and Zambia. *BMJ Open*, 2022. **12**(4): p. e056767.

14. World Health Organization (WHO). Sustainable Management of Radiotherapy Facilities and Equipment. 2023; Available from: https://www.who.int/publications/i/item/9789240075061 [Accessed 2024-12-14].

15. Grossi, R.M., The IAEA's Rays of Hope Leverages Nuclear Science and Collaboration to Fight Cancer in Developing Countries. *J Cancer Policy*, 2022. **34**: p. 100357.

16. Grossi, R.M., Rays of Hope: The IAEA Ups Its Commitment to Cancer Care. *Lancet Oncol*, 2022. **23**(6): p. 702–703.

17. International Atomic Energy Agency (IAEA). Rays of Hope Anchor Centres. [Accessed 2025-01-16]; Available from: https://www.iaea.org/services/rays-of-hope/anchor-centres.

CHAPTER 10

Education and Training Specific to Global Collaborative Activities

Jacob Van Dyk and Akshaya Neil Arya

10.1 CHAPTER OBJECTIVES

- To summarize options for international engagement

- To describe historical context and inequities of past global health relationships

- To address global health obstacles

- To describe the development of partnership programmes

- To highlight training contents for involvement in global activities

- To provide recommendations on education and training considerations to foster successful global collaborative activities.

10.2 INTRODUCTION

While the interest in global health activities (GHAs) among medical students increased dramatically in the early 2000s with the number of medical students participating in global health (GH) electives increasing from 6% in 1996 to 29% in 2014 [1], recent data has shown a decrease from 24% in 2019 to 11% in 2023 in the wake of the pandemic [2]. Participants are

DOI: 10.1201/9781003527749-10

eager to engage in these activities for a variety of reasons, including personal and professional growth, exchange of information, development of cultural competency, desire to reduce health disparities, interest in various cultures, enhancement of their GH competencies prior to graduation, development of lifelong relationships and friendships, a desire to travel, and possible professional advancement and recognition [3–5]. Similar trends are appearing in medical physics and radiation oncology, where residency programmes are promoting international electives [6]. Chapter 2 in this book describes how medical physicists are increasingly involved in global collaborations not only at the educational level, but at any stage of their professional careers with the goal of improving the quality and safety of patient care. The American Association of Physicists in Medicine (AAPM) has restructured organizationally to add an International Council in 2020 to "develop, prioritize, and coordinate international activities of the Corporation, including external collaborations related to international activities." The question is, to what extent are individual medical physicists prepared to take on the challenges associated with international activities?

There are multiple issues that are connected to this question. Indeed, books have been written especially for medical students and also relevant to other healthcare workers, embarking on international health experiences [7, 8]. This chapter highlights issues related to international activities, and the education and training considerations that are helpful for global engagement.

10.3 OPTIONS OF INTERNATIONAL ENGAGEMENT FOR MEDICAL PHYSICISTS

Medical physicists have been involved in a variety of international activities, many of which are analogous to international activities in other healthcare-related professions. These can be summarized as follows and can be categorized into three main topical areas: (1) teaching/training, (2) advising, and (3) partnering.

10.3.1 Teaching/Training

- One-week (or more) professional development courses (or workshops) including both classroom lecturing and hands-on training in the clinical setting, mostly in radiation therapy and imaging departments. Some of these courses are given jointly with radiation oncologists, radiobiologists, or radiology physicians, and/or radiation therapists or diagnostic radiology technologists.

- Training on the use of certain types of techniques or technologies as applied in the clinic for radiotherapy or imaging. These could range from a few days and up.

- Graduate course teaching (master's or PhD level) or residency training in both face-to-face and virtual settings.

10.3.2 Advising

- Advising on setting up a graduate programme (at the MSc or PhD levels).

- Advising on medical physics–related activities for the development of a new radiotherapy or imaging department or centre.

- Advising on international medical physics certification options and procedures.

- Advising on radiation safety issues, especially as related to regulatory requirements, and also for training purposes.

- Reviewing designs/layouts of new radiotherapy or imaging departments.

- Advising on purchase considerations for new technologies.

- Development of national or regional medical physics organizations.

10.3.3 Partnering

- As mentor/mentee (mostly virtually).

- In research projects, both clinically oriented and basic science oriented as related to radiotherapy and imaging.

- In support of commissioning clinical radiation therapy or imaging equipment, or submission of regulatory documentation for radiation safety and licensing procedures, or setting up quality assurance programmes. These could range from a few weeks to a few months or longer, and usually as on-site visits.

10.4 ADDRESSING GLOBAL HEALTH OBSTACLES

An online survey of 264 GH professionals highlighted the significance of GH challenges [9]. Four factors related to the barriers' seriousness were: (1) resource limitations, (2) priority selection (e.g., differences of opinion regarding what should be prioritized), (3) corruption, lack of competence (e.g., obtaining healthcare leadership positions through means other than competence and expertise), and (4) social and cultural barriers. Solutions were suggested for the five most frequently selected barriers, although individual barriers may have different levels of importance for different medical specialties.

10.5 LEARNING FROM MISTAKES OF THE PAST

10.5.1 Colonialism

Colonialism involves one nation having control or influence over another nation and has generally been manifested by a power imbalance between high-income countries (HICs) impacting low- to middle-income countries (LMICs). Similar power asymmetries exist today at the personal level [10] with individuals in HICs feeling that they have the "answer" to the "problems" in LMICs even in the GH context [11]. Do we work together in true, equitable, and mutual partnerships, or do "we" show them how "we" do it? Also, according to Hussain *et al.* [11], GH partnerships that aim to "help" often mirror colonial relationships, with members of HICs being given greater opportunities in LMICs than the other way around. "Global health programs are also known to amplify 'brain drain' rather than nurture 'brain gain.'" The negative impact of globalization should be understood as part of our challenge in participating in GHAs.

10.5.2 Neocolonialism

"The geopolitical practice of using capitalism, business globalization, and cultural imperialism to influence a country, opening their economy to transnational corporations and facilitating the cultural assimilation of the colonised people" [12]. The term was coined by Kwame Nkruma, President of Ghana (1960–1966).

10.5.3 Racism

There is a direct link between colonialism and racism. To quote from the Comment section of *The Lancet*, "The O'Neill–*Lancet* Commission on Racism, Structural Discrimination, and Global Health posits racism as one of the most consequential transnational phenomena to impact the health and lives of afflicted communities globally." We need to be educated about the impact of racialized healthcare disparities by countering existing racist and discriminatory practices and policies.

10.5.4 Decolonizing Global Health

There is a well-recognized scarcity of healthcare workers in LMICs, also in medical physics circles [13, 14]. This has been exacerbated by the migration of healthcare workers from LMICs to HICs and represents a modern version of colonial practice [15]. This *Lancet* editorial provides several recommendations on steps towards decolonization including appropriate funding and building LMIC research capacity. While there are multiple pathways for decolonization, medical physicists should be aware of the issues and be careful to work in full partnership with our LMIC colleagues by humbly asking (rather than telling) how we might be able to contribute to their needs (see Chapter 20 of [8]).

10.6 DEVELOPING PARTNERSHIP PROGRAMMES

The Working Group on Ethics Guidelines for Global Health Training (WEIGHT) developed a set of guidelines for institutions, trainees, and sponsors of field-based GH training on ethics and best practices in this setting [16]. Many of these guidelines are also relevant for partnership activities in the medical physics context. Well-structured partnership programmes are dependent on good communications with a clear outline of expectations and delineation of roles and responsibilities of all parties, budgets, duration of involvement, participation in and distribution of written reports, and other products.

10.7 STANDARDIZING TRAINING FOR INVOLVEMENT IN GLOBAL HEALTH ACTIVITIES

As medical physicists, we have very little formalized training in GH experiences with only a few residency programmes offering GH electives. There is no description of any formalized GH training associated with these electives. Furthermore, many medical physicists involved in GHAs are well beyond the age of undergraduate or graduate training and, thus, are dependent on their own education or on organized continuing medical education activities. The question is what we, as medical physicists, can learn from the GH medical education programmes that are relevant for medical physicists?

Anderson and Bocking [17] helped develop predeparture training guidelines for the Canadian Federation of Medical Students (CFMS), later adopted by the Association of Faculties of Medicine of Canada (AFMC) for GHAs using five subject categories: (1) Personal Health, (2) Travel Safety, (3) Cultural Awareness, (4) Language Competencies, and (5) Ethical Considerations. Note that these were primarily outlined for undergraduate medical students; however, many of the issues are also relevant for medical physics short- and long-term projects around the globe.

10.7.1 Personal Health

Personal health considerations include an understanding of common infections and diseases relevant to the country being visited, including water and food safety, injury prevention especially as related to transportation safety, and vector-borne illness prevention. Immunization requirements vary by country and can be determined through local travel clinics and usually need to be considered two to three months prior to travel. Health travel insurance is a must and should be reviewed for its details. Other issues to be reviewed are dependent on circumstances and include personal protective equipment, HIV pre- and post-exposure prophylaxis, and available access to medical care at the site of the visit should it be needed. Any medications for personal use, such as malaria prophylaxis, should be brought by the incumbent for the length of time as needed.

10.7.2 Travel Safety

Political instability, poorly functioning healthcare systems, and inadequate infrastructures such as roads and various modes of transportation increase the risk of personal injury. Furthermore, visitors from HICs are at risk for theft or being exploited (e.g., taxis, lodging, street vendors, pickpockets). Understanding the risks and circumstances prior to arrival helps mitigate these events. Travel advisory advice provided by the national governments of the incumbent traveller should be reviewed. A documentation of emergency contacts should be recorded prior to travel including the government agencies of the traveller.

10.7.3 Cultural Awareness

Cultural, religious, and gender issues vary dramatically by nation and locale. An understanding of these issues prior to travel aids in identifying power imbalances and adaptation to appropriate communications in terms of mannerisms and speech. It is helpful to understand gender and cultural issues to aid in increasing efficiency, quality, and sustainability of the work of the collaborative initiative. Allison and Whaling [18] refer to this as "cultural competence." For example, in some cultures, it is inappropriate for men and women who are not related or married to be seen together in a social situation. This may impact decisions on where you will sit in a meeting room, whether to get on an elevator, or deciding on who you will have a coffee or a meal with [18]. In some contexts, homosexuality is illegal and could be persecuted. These considerations are not only relevant for the visitor but could have a significant impact (perhaps even more so) on the local collaborators. Food, drink, and clothing all have their cultural nuances. Alcohol is taboo in some circles and is encouraged in other social settings. In some cultures, how we dress is significant, especially when it is important to dress modestly with shoulders and knees covered, perhaps with long sleeves, long trousers for men, and long skirts for women.

Religious perspectives could have an impact on healthcare delivery and care seeking, in addition to how one seeks employment and how one is promoted. In some instances, workplace hierarchy is determined by gender or age and not necessarily by expertise. Furthermore, the profession of medical physics is viewed in different ways in different countries. It is important to recognize differences in perspective but not allow them to generate barriers.

Norms related to space, privacy, and confidentiality also have their cultural nuances. The perception of time and scheduling with its rigidity in the Global North could be very different in other cultures where a social hierarchical order of arrival might be of greater importance. To avoid culture shock, preparation in advance is key. It is important "to develop a sense of cultural humility that enables us to be not only competent but receptive and collaborative" [18].

10.7.4 Language/Communication Competencies

There are both similarities and significant differences in terms of communication issues for short- and long-term GHAs of medical physicists in comparison to medical residents or medical undergraduate student placements. One of the main differences is that medical practitioners communicate directly with the patient. Medical physicists are involved in high-tech activities and only for special procedures communicate with the patient directly. Most of the communication involves local medical physicists, medical doctors, other science-related experts, or administrators, all of whom will have a university education, often (although not always) with a foreign language requirement. However, developing good communication remains a challenge to be overcome.

Verbal and nonverbal communications vary from culture to culture. For example, head movement is commonly used to communicate positive versus negative responses. In the North American context, vertical head movement denotes positivity while in Bulgaria, this response pattern is reversed and vertical head movement means "no" [19]. Considerations in this context include that organizers of the GHAs select participants, if possible, who are from the diaspora of the country being visited and to gain as much insight into issues related to nonverbal communication as possible to avoid being exposed to unwanted circumstances.

Some business leaders have divided styles of communication into "transactional" versus "interactional." The distinction between the two styles is summarized in Table 10.1. Transaction deals with the task at hand and is intended to get the job done quickly. Interaction occurs when two people are engaged socially and actively participating in the process to get the job done. The tendency is that those in the Global North are more transactional while those in the Global South are more interactional. Interactional connections are likely to have better results in the long run [20].

10.7.5 Ethical Considerations

Ethical considerations are addressed in detail in Chapter 15, including the four principles of justice, beneficence, nonmaleficence, and autonomy. However, Pinto and Upshur [21] note that these four principles may be interpreted differently according to the cultural context and describe the following four additional concepts useful in GH work.

TABLE 10.1   Styles of Communication

Transactional	Interactional
• Business driven	• Relationship building
• To the point	• Check-in, e.g., How are you?
• Get the job done	• About the person
• Short-term thinking	• Service driven
• Basic/mechanical communication	• Conversational
	• Engaging
	• Provide a sense of belonging

1. Humility: GH workers need to recognize their own limitations and realize that their training in the developed world does not necessarily translate to competence in all healthcare settings. "Humility is crucial and helps undermine neocolonial trends that often permeate relationships between the North and South."

2. Introspection: A rigorous examination of one's motives is of great importance along with an awareness of one's privilege. Pintos and Ross provide a set of questions for medical students [21]. These questions are included in Table 10.3 in the "Recommendations" section of this chapter.

3. Solidarity: The GH worker should ensure their goals and values are aligned with the community where they aim to work, in both clinical and research settings. "True solidarity exists when citizens of the community are mobilized, when capacity building of local organizations and strengthened links within civil society occurs, and when attempts are made to bridge power imbalances between the wealthy and the poor."

4. Social justice: "Ultimately global health work should be concerned with diminishing the gross inequity seen in the world" [21]. This could mean going further "upstream" from what they see and consider the underlying causes of ill health.

Larson *et al.* [22] have developed a user-friendly equity tool for valuing a global health partnership using a simple questionnaire to cultivate equity in each unique context.

10.8 CODE OF CONDUCT

A code of conduct (or code of practice) is generally defined as a set of rules that members of an organization or people with a particular job or position must follow [23]. While these "rules" are multidimensional, most are common sense. Table 10.2 summarizes some examples.

The last item in Table 10.2 requires some further comments. Doobay-Persaud *et al.* [24] explain clearly the consequences of performing outside scope of training (POST), at least for medical practitioners [24]. However, the issues are relevant for medical physicists as well. For example, if we, from the Global North, are present without an oncologist, we might be asked a clinical question for which we are not formally trained. Or, we

TABLE 10.2   Examples of Code of Conduct "Rules" Relevant for Medical Physicists

- Always be courteous and on time
- Engage with participants
- Do not pretend to know it all
- Adapt to language concerns (e.g., pace and clarity of speaking)
- Be flexible, adapt to circumstances
- Respect and mutuality (e.g., learn from each other)
- Do not assume (e.g., language, technical issues, knowledge skills). Find out!
- Do not practice outside scope of training (POST)

might be asked about therapy or imaging machine repairs, which in our own circumstances would be handled by electronics service personnel. Clear responses need to address only the issues for which we have been formally trained.

10.9 SUMMARY AND RECOMMENDATIONS

10.9.1 Summary

Global health involves social, political, economic, environmental, and cultural considerations, especially as they relate to healthcare. Most medical physicists have had no education or training to address the multiple complex factors involved in international collaborations. This chapter has outlined many of these considerations and makes it clear that some form of education and training is essential for GHAs to achieve the desired results, both for effectiveness and sustainability. The following recommendations provide a foundational framework for participating in GHAs. These recommendations are strongly influenced by *The Practitioner's Guide to Global Health*, which describes an interactive massive open online course (MOOC) specially made for physicians in training [25], although adapted for medical physicists. Note that the preparation needs of international learners rotating to HICs are not the same as those of US learners rotating to LMICs [25]. The recommendations may also be relevant for other professionals travelling abroad for collaborative purposes, especially those in fields connected with medical physics.

10.9.2 Recommendations

1. Education and training for all those involved in GHAs are essential for adequate preparation for safe, effective, and sustainable results [23].

2. The contents of this education and training should include the topics and objectives described in Table 10.3 as summarized from the literature [7, 21–23] and adapted for medical physicists.

TABLE 10.3 Education and Training Topics as Determined from the Literature and Adapted for Medical Physicists [7, 21–23]

The Big Picture (Before the GHA)

1	Describe and prioritize your objectives and motivation, both personal and structural, and short-term and long-term, for undertaking a GHA.
2	What are the benefits and who will receive them, and what are the costs and who will bear them?
3	In the context of very limited resources for GH needs, is your work feasible, cost-effective, necessary, focused, and justified? What exists close-by?
4	Will it work to undermine disparity or actually contribute to it? Will there be a net benefit to the community? Use the equity tool [22] for guidance in GH partnerships.
5	What do you hope to bring back to your community, and with whom will you share it?
6	Is your work sustainable, and if not, will this leave a negative impact?
7	Differentiate between different types of GHAs and determine which ones provide the best fit for you.
8	Analyze factors including timing, duration, and location to plan an appropriate GHA.
9	What do you need to do to prepare for your work, both practical and personal?
10	Develop a plan to address logistical issues including personal, health, and security concerns that affect successful completion of a GHA.
11	Identify and describe options for funding and budgeting for a GHA.

Preparation on the Ground (Before and During GHA)

1	Be clear about communication contacts and lines of authority of the institution/organization being visited.
2	Establish the particulars of project-related departmental technologies in use or to be installed. Include the details (e.g., make, model, specifications) of all ancillary devices that are likely to be used during the visit.
3	Develop a written agreement about the terms of the project. Ensure that this is signed by the appropriate responsible persons recognizing that this may have greater weight in some cultures and contexts versus others.

(Continued)

TABLE 10.3   (*Continued*)

4	Effectively prepare for and arrange airport transportation and travel documents for a smooth arrival.
5	Improve cultural awareness and security preparedness in the areas of communication, transportation, housing, insurance, money, clothing, and evacuation.
6	Identify proper vaccinations and medications to minimize health hazards.
7	Prepare an appropriately inclusive yet "light" packing list that ensures preparation for emergencies and environmental exposures.
8	Describe practical strategies for an enriched GHA that benefits you and your host community.
9	Navigate and manage personal and family responsibilities.
10	Identify and avoid common medical issues that you may encounter on the ground.
11	Recognize personal and property safety risks, including risks related to transportation and to drug and alcohol consumption.
12	Identify professional, ethical, and cultural issues you may encounter.
13	Practice within your scope of training.
14	Use various modes of communication, including social media, responsibly.

Reflection (After GHA)

1	Identify and explain components of "reverse culture shock" upon returning from a GHA.
2	Identify strategies for effectively "reintegrating" into your home and work life upon returning from a GHA.
3	Effectively deal with potential health issues upon returning from a GHA.
4	Effectively advocate for other individuals at your institution or within your organization to identify medical physics opportunities, educational opportunities, and funding structures for future GHAs.

Note: GHA, global health activity; GH, global health.

REFERENCES

1. Goller, T.M., A.; Moore, M.; Dougherty A., Pre-Departure Training for Global Health Electives at US Medical Schools. *Medical Science Education*, 2017. **27**: p. 535–541.
2. Association of American Medical Colleges (AAMC). Medical School Graduation Questionnaire: 2023 All Schools Summary Report. 2023 [cited 2024 06 October 2024].
3. Connor, S.E.J., L.J.; Covvey,J.R.; Kahaleh, A.A.; Park, S.K.; Ryan, M.; Klein-Fedyshin, M.; Goldchin, N.; Veillard, R.B., A Systematic Review of Global Health Assessment for Education in Healthcare Professions. *Annals of Global Health*, 2022. **88**(1): p. 1–49.
4. Arya, N. and K. Chan, Should I Stay or Should I Go? And What can I Do When I Get There?, in *Preparing for International Health Experiences: A Practical Guide*, A.N. Arya, Editor. 2017, Routledge: New York. p. 13–20.
5. Van Dyk, J., D. Jaffray, and R. Jeraj, Global Considerations for the Practice of Medical Physics in Radiation Oncology, in *The Modern Technology of Radiation Oncology: A Compendium for Medical Physicists and Radiation Oncologists*, J. Van Dyk, Editor. 2020, Medical Physics Publishing: Madison, WI. p. 437–458.
6. Brown, D.W., *et al.*, The Case for Elective International Residency Rotations. *International Journal of Radiation Oncology, Biology, Physics*, 2015. **93**(5): p. 963–964.
7. Arya, A.N., *Preparing for International Health Experiences: A Practical Guide*. 2017, New York: Routledge.
8. Arya, A.N. and J. Evert, *Global Health Experiential Education: From Theory to Practice*. 2018, New York: Routledge.
9. Weiss, B. and A.A. Pollack, Barriers to Global Health Development: An International Quantitative Survey. *PLoS One*, 2017. **12**(10): p. e0184846.
10. Finkel, M.L., *et al.*, What Do Global Health Practitioners Think about Decolonizing Global Health? *Annals of Global Health*, 2022. **88**(1): p. 61.
11. Hussain, M., *et al.*, Colonization and Decolonization of Global Health: Which Way Forward? *Global Health Action*, 2023. **16**(1): p. 2186575.
12. Oguejiofor, W.O., The Interrelationships between Western Imperialism and Underdevelopment in Africa. *Arts Social Science Journal*, 2015. **6**(3): p. 1000112.
13. Atun, R., *et al.*, Expanding Global Access to Radiotherapy. *Lancet Oncology*, 2015. **16**(10): p. 1153–1186.
14. Hricak, H., *et al.*, Medical Imaging and Nuclear Medicine: A Lancet Oncology Commission. *Lancet Oncology*, 2021. **22**(4): p. e136–e172.
15. Erondu, N.A., et al., Towards Anti-Racist Policies and Strategies to Reduce Poor Health Outcomes in Racialised Communities: Introducing the O'Neill-Lancet Commission on Racism, Structural Discrimination, and Global Health. *Lancet*, 2023. **401**(10391): p. 1834–1836.

16. Crump, J.A., J. Sugarman, and Working Group on Ethics Guidelines for Global Health Training, Ethics and best practice guidelines for training experiences in global health. *American Journal of Tropical Medicine and Hygiene*, 2010. **83**(6): p. 1178–1182.
17. Anderson, K. and N. Bocking. Preparing Medical Students for Electives in Low-Resource Settings: A Template for National Guidelines for Pre-Departure Training. 2008 [Accessed 2025-01-01]; Available from: https://www.cfms.org/files/GH-report-documents/resource-documents/Pre-Departure%20Guidelines%20Final.pdf.
18. Allison, J. and M. Whaling, Seeking Cultural Competence, in *Preparing for International Health Experiences: A Practical Guide*, A.N. Arya, Editor. 2017, Routledge: New York.
19. Andonova, E. and H.A. Taylor, Nodding in Dis/Agreement: A Tale of Two Cultures. *Cognitive Processing*, 2012. **13 Suppl 1**: p. S79-S82.
20. Richards, J.C. Teaching Speaking for Interactional versus Transactional Purposes. [Accessed 2025-01-10]; Available from: https://www.professorjackrichards.com/teaching-speaking-interactional-versus-transactional-purposes/.
21. Pinto, A.D. and R.E. Upshur, Global Health Ethics for Students. *Developing World Bioethics*, 2009. **9**(1): p. 1-10.
22. Larson, C.P., et al., The Equity Tool for Valuing Global Health Partnerships. *Global Health: Science and Practice*, 2022. **10**(2): e2100316.
23. Cambridge Dictionary. *Code of Conduct*. 23 October 2024]; Available from: https://dictionary.cambridge.org/dictionary/english/code-of-conduct.
24. Doobay-Persaud, A., *et al.*, Extent, Nature and Consequences of Performing Outside Scope of Training in Global Health. *Global Health*, 2019. **15**(1): p. 60.
25. Jacquet, G.A., *et al.*, The Practitioner's Guide to Global Health: An Interactive, Online, Open-Access Curriculum Preparing Medical Learners for Global Health Experiences. *Medical Education Online*, 2018. **23**(1): p. 1503914.

CHAPTER 11

Advocacy and Science Diplomacy in Support of International Collaborations

Eva Bezak, Loredana Marcu, and
Ana Maria Marques da Silva

11.1 CHAPTER OBJECTIVES

- To define advocacy, diplomacy, and science diplomacy
- To describe the need for advocacy and diplomacy
- To describe the applications of advocacy and diplomacy in science and medical physics
- To review the challenges and benefits of advocacy and diplomacy in medical physics
- To provide recommendations in support of advocacy and diplomacy activities for successful global medical physics collaborations

11.2 INTRODUCTION

In medical physics, we often understand the role of the medical physics profession in terms of equipment commissioning, radiation safety, quality

DOI: 10.1201/9781003527749-11

assurance, and healthcare delivery, as well as research and development. Perhaps it is not immediately obvious how medical physicists contribute more broadly to science diplomacy and advocacy, facilitation of international collaborations, international education, or equipment support programmes that ultimately inform governments and policy-makers, improve the standard of the profession, and contribute towards improving the equity of healthcare and access around the world. After providing a basic definition of science diplomacy and advocacy, this chapter discusses examples of medical physics initiatives in this space. There is ample evidence that professional organizations, such as those in the field of medical physics (e.g., the International Organization for Medical Physics (IOMP), or the International Union for Physical and Engineering Sciences in Medicine (IUPESM)), play important intellectual, material, and social roles in international communities [1, 2]. The practical examples provided here focus on Europe and North and South Americas as examples of high-income and low- to middle-income economies in which medical physics is practised.

Advocacy involves promoting or defending a particular cause or policy, typically through public support, lobbying, and education. In the context of medical physics, advocacy encompasses efforts to highlight the importance of the field, influence policy, and secure resources for research and clinical applications [3].

Diplomacy is the practice of managing international relations and negotiations to achieve mutually beneficial outcomes. In medical physics, diplomacy fosters collaborations and agreements between countries and organizations to advance the field globally.

Science Diplomacy "is a novel field of research and translational practice that employs integration of science and technology and international collaborations to address the big questions that mankind faces globally" [4]. While various national and international policies or guidelines should be based on community consultation, ultimately, all decisions must also be informed by scientific facts and evidence, as appropriate.

11.2.1 The Need for Advocacy and Diplomacy

Advocacy and diplomacy are crucial for advancing medical physics internationally for several reasons:

1. **Recognition and Visibility**: Despite its critical role in healthcare, medical physics often lacks the recognition it deserves. Advocacy is essential for raising awareness about the field's contributions to cancer treatment, diagnostic imaging, and radiation safety. By actively promoting the profession, medical physicists can ensure their expertise is valued and integrated into healthcare policies and practices [5].

2. **Coordination and Collaboration**: A lack of coordination and awareness can hinder international collaborations in medical physics. Advocacy helps bridge these gaps by promoting global standards and practices, fostering communication between organizations, and encouraging joint research initiatives. Diplomacy plays a role in negotiating partnerships and agreements that facilitate these collaborations.

3. **Funding and Resources**: Medical physics research and clinical applications potentially require significant funding and resources. Advocacy can influence policy-makers and funding bodies to allocate necessary research and technology development resources. Diplomacy can help in securing international funding and support for global projects.

4. **Education and Training**: Advocacy is necessary to address medical physicists' educational and training needs nationally and globally [5]. This includes promoting the importance of specialized training programmes and professional development opportunities. Diplomacy can aid in establishing international training programmes and exchanges that enhance the skills of medical physicists worldwide.

5. **Policy and Regulation**: Medical physicists often face challenges related to regulatory frameworks and policy. Advocacy can help shape policies that support the field, while diplomacy can facilitate discussions between countries to harmonize regulations and standards.

Some applications of advocacy and diplomacy in medical physics are collated in Table 11.1, while Table 11.2 presents the main challenges and benefits of advocacy and diplomacy in this field.

The following sections illustrate some applications and challenges of advocacy and science diplomacy in medical physics across Europe and

TABLE 11.1   Applications of Advocacy and Diplomacy in Medical Physics

Advocacy Activities

Task	Role	Activities
Organizing	Building a strong community of medical physicists and supporters.	Forming professional associations, organizing conferences, and creating platforms for sharing knowledge and experiences.
Education and awareness	Educating legislators, healthcare professionals, and the public about the role of medical physics.	Providing information on radiation protection, advanced diagnostic and treatment modalities, and the impact of medical physics on patient care.
Research and policy	Advocating for increased funding for research and development in medical physics.	Lobbying for policy changes and engaging with policy-makers to highlight the benefits of investing in medical physics.
Regulatory efforts	Working with regulatory bodies to ensure that standards and guidelines reflect the latest advancements in medical physics.	Contributing to the development of safety protocols and best practices.

Diplomacy Activities

Task	Role	Activities
International collaborations	Establishing partnerships between countries, organizations, and industry to enhance research capabilities and share knowledge.	Working with international bodies such as the International Atomic Energy Agency (IAEA), the International Organization for Medical Physics (IOMP), and the World Health Organization (WHO) [6].
Negotiations and agreements	Facilitate cross-border research, technology transfer, and educational exchanges.	Formal agreements between institutions and countries that support collaborative projects and mutual benefits.
Cultural and linguistic considerations	Understanding and addressing cultural and linguistic barriers that may impact international collaborations.	Fostering a respectful and inclusive environment for diverse stakeholders [7].

TABLE 11.2   Main Challenges and Benefits of Advocacy and Diplomacy in Medical Physics

Challenges Type	Premise/Description	Addressing the Challenge
Diverse needs and priorities	Medical physics is practised in various contexts worldwide, from highly advanced to under-resourced settings.	Tailored advocacy strategies and diplomatic approaches that consider local conditions and priorities, while aiming to harmonize the profession.
Limited recognition	The lack of recognition of medical physics as a distinct and essential profession can hinder advocacy efforts.	Sustained efforts to demonstrate the field's value and impact on healthcare.
Resource constraints	Advocacy and diplomatic activities often require significant resources, including time, funding, and expertise.	Increase resources to not restrict the scope and effectiveness of these efforts.
Cultural and linguistic barriers	International collaborations can be complicated by differences in language, culture, and healthcare practices.	Navigating these differences and fostering mutual understanding.
Benefits Type	**Premise/Description**	**Benefit/Outcome**
Enhanced global collaboration	Advocacy and diplomacy can lead to strengthened international collaborations, resulting in shared knowledge, resources, and best practices.	Accelerate advancements in medical physics and improve patient outcomes globally.
Increased visibility and recognition	Advocacy and diplomacy lead to a better understanding by the government and public of the medical physics profession and its contribution.	Medical physicists and their organizations are seen as major partners for planning current and future healthcare, radiation safety standards, artificial intelligence (AI) implementation, and more.
Increased funding and support	Successful advocacy can result in increased funding and support for medical physics research and education.	Increased innovation and improved quality of care in various healthcare settings.
Improved standards and policies	Advocacy can influence the development of better standards and policies in medical physics,	Improved safety, efficacy, and patient care.
Professional development	International collaborations and advocacy efforts can provide opportunities for professional development and training.	Enhanced skills and expertise of medical physicists. Harmonized professional standards across the world,

America and issues reported by medical physics communities from other parts of the world.

11.3 APPLICATIONS OF ADVOCACY AND SCIENCE DIPLOMACY IN MEDICAL PHYSICS ACROSS THE WORLD

11.3.1 The European Scenario

Scientific advances and professional developments in medical physics are facilitated by collaborations, whether on a national or international level. In view of this, a good model for advocacy and science diplomacy in medical physics is the European Federation of Organisations for Medical Physics (EFOMP), which is an umbrella organization for all National Member Organisations (NMOs), currently encompassing 37 European countries with over 9200 medical physicists [8]. One of the six governing committees of EFOMP is the European and International Matters Committee, with its primary responsibilities to represent the interests of EFOMP to European and international bodies related to medical physics, to formulate proposals addressed to relevant bodies of the European Union (such as the European Parliament and Commission) on issues in medical physics, and to liaise with European and international organizations through various professional activities for the common benefit of medical physicists. Consequently, these collective goals of the member countries envisage both scientific and educational collaborations across borders as well as political and legislative ones to strengthen the position of the medical physics profession among other healthcare occupations.

Some of the most successful activities towards advocacy and science diplomacy are undertaken through working groups and special interest groups under EFOMP's umbrella. To date, a significant number of working groups in several medical physics-related subfields have been established that incorporate experts and consultants throughout Europe to fill in either scientific, logistic, or legislative gaps in specific areas, e.g., development of quality control protocol for angiographic and fluoroscopic systems, dosimetry in molecular radiotherapy, the role of the medical physicist in clinical trials, medical physics education for the non-physics healthcare professions, breast tomosynthesis quality control protocol, and so on. Many of these working groups achieved the creation and publication of policy statements to be used as guidelines, particularly by member countries that lack an appropriate legislative framework regarding education and training in medical physics [9–11]. Furthermore, to provide all European countries (and others) with learning guidelines for medical physicists, core curricula in all medical physics fields (radiology/imaging, radiotherapy, nuclear medicine) are being developed by experts in the field and disseminated [11]. Also, several working groups were created in joint ventures with the American Association of Physicists in Medicine (AAPM), leading to valuable documents that assist medical physicists worldwide in their daily undertakings [12, 13].

Special interest groups (SIG) established within EFOMP bring together medical physicists from all European countries to offer an interactive professional platform related to an area of interest or group of professionals. The newest and very successful SIG is related to early career professionals, who play a vital role in the evolution of our profession. As young physicists require motivation and a suitable environment to develop, EFOMP has created an official platform for learning and education, and professional networking, covering all aspects of the profession [14]. Since the formation of the SIG, several workshops and webinars have been organized by and for the young physicists to stimulate the development of highly desirable soft skills, including strategic planning, communication, and pedagogical skills, while encouraging team building [15]. Mentorship across borders is currently being implemented as an additional aid to young physicists' professional and scientific developments (see Chapter 8). It is anticipated that the involvement of young researchers in science diplomacy on medical physics will stimulate collaborations between low- and high-income countries and accelerate professional mobilities across Europe. This would encourage more rapid employment of a unified training and education programme in medical physics, which is one of EFOMP's key goals, together with the recognition by the European Commission of the Medical Physics Expert nomenclature across Europe.

11.3.2 The American Scenario

The largest national medical physics society in the world, with almost 10,000 members, the American Association of Physicists in Medicine (AAPM) persevered in developing targeted marketing, advocacy, and communication tools to articulate value-based medical physics effectively. Several actions show the importance of advocacy for the association, such as the AAPM Government Relations Office, which works in conjunction with the AAPM Government and Regulatory Affairs Committee (GRAC), following legislative activities that may impact the practice of medical physicists (licensing or credentialing) and influence professional requirements in the field. They also lobby by appointing AAPM members in congressional hearings and setting up meetings with legislators. Beyond the political actors, AAPM advocacy actions work through formal cooperation between AAPM and other medical organizations, such as the American College of Radiology (ACR), the American College of Radiation Oncology (ACRO), the American Society for Radiation Oncology (ASTRO), and the American Academy of Health Physics (AAHP). A notable result of the collaborative effort between organizations was the publication of the MIPPA (Medical Care Improvements for Providers and Protection Act) law in 2008, where the accreditation requirement of CT, MR, and PET scanners in outpatient centres included an annual inspection by medical physicists. A joint commission expanded the requirements for outpatient and hospital locations, improving patient safety and care, and increasing the opportunities for imaging medical physicists.

Another significant result was the approval of the CARE Act 2011 (Consistency, Accuracy, Responsibility, and Excellence (CARE) in Medical Imaging and Radiation Therapy Act) in the US House of Representatives, which ensures the safety of patients receiving potentially life-saving radiation therapy procedures by setting minimum certification and educational standards for non-physician technical personnel performing imaging and administering radiation therapy.

In 2020, AAPM created the Smart Advocacy Subcommittee under the Professional Council to defend medical physics with all stakeholders, from industry to government. This subcommittee plays a vital role in advocating for the function and activities of medical physics to non-physicist professionals, legislators, administrators, physicians, and patients. The subcommittee coordinates, informs, and summarizes advocacy initiatives for AAPM members, engages the public through lectures and education at festivals, TEDx Talks, public events, and develops advocacy training for medical physicists.

In Brazil, since the end of the 1990s, medical physicists have been enrolled in constructing rules, guidelines, and legislation about the medical imaging and therapy equipment that uses radiation. In cooperation with governmental entities, such as the Brazilian Health Regulatory Agency (ANVISA) and the National Commission of Nuclear Energy (CNEN), representatives from the Brazilian Association of Medical Physics (ABFM) helped to build the primary legislation regarding the use of radiation in imaging and therapy in medicine. In 1998, the first Brazilian federal law was approved [16] to rule the use of medical equipment emitting ionizing radiation, guiding the authorization and commissioning of imaging departments, especially in quality assurance and radiation protection aspects. In 2019 and 2022, the Brazilian federal government updated and published the regulations for ionizing radiation quality control and equipment performance limits in all medical imaging modalities and extended them to ensure the inclusion of non-ionizing imaging modalities, such as ultrasound and magnetic resonance imaging [17]. In parallel, CNEN published the Brazilian requirements for radiation protection and quality assurance in radiation therapy and nuclear medicine operations, establishing the minimum requirements regarding organizational infrastructure, staff, radiation protection processes and devices, and quality assurance procedures [18].

One of Latin America's most organized advocacy political movements occurred in Brazil in 2012 when ABFM representatives and scholars went to the Brazilian House of Representatives and the Ministry of Health to advocate for recognizing medical physicists as health professionals. In 2013, the Brazilian Ministry of Health and Ministry of Education authorized and started funding scholarships for two years (5760 hours) of medical physics residency programmes for clinical training with the same full-time salary as medical residents [16].

As previously mentioned, advocacy should be conducted through formal representatives as well as through communication actions. In 2016, the AAPM launched the initiative Medical Physics 3.0 (MP3.0), which has led to a web presence [19] offering content including Good Practices, Areas of Growth Opportunities, Inspiring Stories, and commissioned videos oriented towards medical physicists and prospective students.

Communication between medical physicists and the public in Latin America improved by creating scientific and professional journals, with papers published in Portuguese, Spanish, and English covering medical physics research, clinical, and professional topics. In collaboration with other medical societies, specific medical physics tracks are included in nuclear medicine, radiology, and radiation oncology meetings, showing the interdisciplinary collaboration between medical physicists and physicians.

11.4 CHALLENGES OF ADVOCACY AND SCIENCE DIPLOMACY IN MEDICAL PHYSICS

Considering the high demand for mobility of medical physicists worldwide, particularly among early career researchers, perhaps one of the biggest challenges facing the profession is the lack of a uniform educational and professional framework for the recognition of the medical physics expert (MPE). In Europe, professional organizations are working with national/governmental administrations to map the regulatory framework for implementing a joint training platform. This action requires high-level diplomatic skills to approach competent authorities and advocacy to promote the growing need for mapping our profession.

The American continent faces similar challenges. While Latin America does not have a standardized curriculum in medical physics, professional societies have regular procedures to certify clinical medical physics experts and to accredit medical physics education and training institutions, ensuring the qualification of these professionals. In Brazil, the MPE certification, organized and led by ABFM, is highly valued or even mandatory for clinical positions, especially when explicitly indicated in rules and legislation. Medical physics positions in public hospitals in Brazil, funded by the local government, require or prefer MPE certification in all medical physics specialties. In other Latin American countries where the national organization does not certify medical physicists or accredit residency programmes, the IOMP is working to satisfy the highest standards established with other international organizations to ensure the quality of medical physics programmes. Another organization serving in this space is the International Medical Physics Certification Board (IMPCB) that has developed and runs a certification programme that (a) meets IOMP guidelines and (b) provides accreditation assessment for countries where the certification programme is not present and/or lacking. In recent years, one medical physics residency programme in Argentina and one master's degree programme in medical physics in Colombia were accredited [20].

Besides education and training, scientific research is another key component of a profession's development. While Horizon Europe is the EU's essential funding programme for research and innovation, statistics show significant discrepancies between grant applications across European countries [21]. As an umbrella organization for all national members, EFOMP is encouraging equitable collaborations among all NMOs to diminish discrepancies regarding involvement in research projects between some Eastern European countries and the rest of Europe. Furthermore, the organization strives to reach a balanced distribution of members from all four corners of Europe in all scientific and educational projects that EFOMP is part of. Science diplomacy should, therefore, be embodied as a critical feature of any medical physics organization, whether national or international, to adequately represent its members and assist the profession on all levels of its development.

11.5 SUMMARY AND RECOMMENDATIONS

11.5.1 Summary

Medical physicists often contribute broadly to science diplomacy and advocacy, facilitation of international collaborations, international education, or equipment support programmes that ultimately inform governments and policymakers, improve the standard of the profession, and contribute towards improving the equity of healthcare and access around the world. Having defined science diplomacy and advocacy, examples are provided of medical physics initiatives in this space. There is ample evidence that professional medical physics organizations play important intellectual, material, and social roles in international communities. The practical examples provided focus on Europe, and North and South Americas, and recognize high-income and low- to middle-income economies in which medical physics is practised.

11.5.2 Recommendations for Successful Global Medical Physics Collaborations

1. **Strengthen Advocacy Networks**: Develop and expand advocacy networks to build a strong, united voice for medical physics. This includes forming alliances with professional organizations, patient groups, and policy-makers to amplify advocacy efforts.

2. **Promote International Dialogues**: Facilitate international dialogues and conferences to foster collaboration and knowledge exchange. This can help address global challenges, share best practices, and develop joint initiatives.

3. **Enhance Training and Education**: Invest in advocacy and diplomacy training for medical physicists to equip them with the skills to promote the field and effectively engage with international stakeholders.

4. **Address Cultural and Linguistic Barriers**: Develop strategies to address cultural and linguistic differences in international collaborations. This includes providing translation services, cultural competency training, and fostering an inclusive environment.

5. **Leverage Technology and Media**: Utilize technology and media platforms to raise awareness about medical physics and its contributions. This includes using social media, online resources, and virtual conferences to reach a global audience.

6. **Foster Inclusivity and Diversity**: Promote inclusivity and diversity in advocacy and diplomatic efforts. This includes addressing gender disparities and ensuring representation from various regions and backgrounds in international collaborations [22].

7. Serve on **Advisory Boards and Governmental Commissions:** This is an important way to safeguard the participation of medical physicists in all activities pertaining to their profession to ensure a high standard of quality assurance across all subfields of medical physics. It is helpful for medical physicists to venture outside the clinical rooms into the world of management, policies, international collaborations, and diplomacy.

REFERENCES

1. Frickel, S., Just science? Organizing scientist activism in the US environmental justice movement. *Sci. Culture*, 2004. **13**(4): p. 449–469.
2. Tormos-Aponte, F., *et al.*, Pathways for diversifying and enhancing science advocacy. *Sci Adv*, 2023. **9**(20): p. eabq4899.
3. Jessani, N.S., *et al.*, Advocacy, activism, and lobbying: How variations in interpretation affects ability for academia to engage with public policy. *PLOS Glob Public Health*, 2022. **2**(3): p. e0000034.
4. Bezak, E., *et al.*, Science diplomacy in medical physics – an international perspective. *Health Technol (Berl)*, 2023. **13**(3): p. 495–503.
5. Bezak, E., J. Damilakis, and M.M. Rehani, Global status of medical physics human resource – the IOMP survey report. *Phys Med*, 2023. **113**: p. 102670.
6. Rehani, M.M., *et al.*, The International Organization for Medical Physics – a driving force for the global development of medical physics. *Health Technol (Berl)*, 2022. **12**(3): p. 617–631.
7. Santos, J.C., *et al.*, Leadership and mentoring in medical physics: the experience of a medical physics international mentoring program. *Phys Med*, 2020. **76**: p. 337–344.
8. European Federation of Organisations for Medical Physics (EFOMP). Available from: https://www.efomp.org. [Accessed 2024-12-31]
9. Caruana, C.J., *et al.*, EFOMP policy statement 18: medical physics education for the non-physics healthcare professions. *Phys Med*, 2023. **111**: p. 102602.
10. Caruana, C.J., *et al.*, EFOMP policy statement 16: The role and competences of medical physicists and medical physics experts under 2013/59/EURATOM. *Phys Med*, 2018. **48**: p. 162–168.
11. Garibaldi, C., et al., The 3(rd) ESTRO-EFOMP core curriculum for medical physics experts in radiotherapy. *Radiother Oncol*, 2022. **170**: p. 89–94.
12. AAPM report no 246, Estimating patient organ dose with computed tomography: a review of present methodology and required DICOM information. 2019.

13. Sechopoulos, I., *et al.*, Joint AAPM Task Group 282/EFOMP Working Group Report: breast dosimetry for standard and contrast-enhanced mammography and breast tomosynthesis. *Med Phys*, 2024. **51**(2): p. 712–739.
14. Marcu, L.G., *et al.*, Early career medical physicist groups in Europe: An EFOMP survey. *Phys Med*, 2022. **95**: p. 89–93.
15. Caruana, C.J. and J. Damilakis, Being an excellent scientist is not enough to succeed! Soft skills for medical physicists. *Eur J Radiol*, 2022. **155**: p. 110108.
16. Brasil. Ministério da Saúde. Secretaria de Vigilância Sanitária. Portaria SVS/MS N° 453, de 1 de Junho de 1998. Available at: https://www.saude.mg .gov.br/images/documentos/Portaria_453.pdf [Accessed 2024-12-25].
17. Brasil. Ministério da Saúde, Agência Nacional de Vigilância Sanitária, Diretoria Colegiada. Resolução – RDC n° 611, de 09 de março de 2022. Brasil: Diário Oficial da União, 2022, p. 107–110. Available at: https://antigo .anvisa.gov.br/documents/10181/6407467/RDC_611_2022_.pdf/c552d93f -b80d-408e-92a0-9fa3573f6d46 [Accessed 2024-12-25].
18. Freitas, M.B. and R.A. Terini, A Formação em Física Médica no Brasil e no Mundo: da Graduação à Pós-graduação. *Rev Bras Fís Méd*, 2019. 13(1).
19. Medical Physics 3.0 (MP3.0). Available at: "https://mp30.aapm.org/" [Accessed 2024-12-25].
20. International Organization of Medical Physics. Accreditation. Available at: https://www.iomp.org/accreditation/.
21. European Court of Auditors, Measures to widen participation in Horizon 2020 were well designed but sustainable change will mostly depend on efforts by national authorities. Available at: https://op.europa.eu/webpub/ eca/special-reports/h2020-15-2022/en/ [Accessed 2024-12-25].
22. Barabino, G., *et al.*, Solutions to gender balance in STEM fields through support, training, education and mentoring: report of the international women in medical physics and biomedical engineering task group. *Sci Eng Ethics*, 2020. **26**(1): p. 275–292.

CHAPTER 12

The Role of Information Computer Technologies (ICTs) and Artificial Intelligence (AI) in Global Collaborations*

Jacob Van Dyk and Issam El Naqa

12.1 CHAPTER OBJECTIVES*

The goal of this chapter is to explore the increasingly important role of information and communication technologies (ICTs) and artificial intelligence (AI) in global collaborations, particularly in the context of medical physics. The following objectives will be addressed:

1. To describe the use of ICTs for global collaborations

2. To describe the applications of AI in global collaborations

3. To suggest minimal requirements for success in global ICT and AI applications

4. To discuss the applications, barriers, and limitations of ICTs and AI in the global context

5. To provide recommendations regarding the use of ICTs and AI for enhancing global applications

---

* For this chapter, it is important to read Section 12.A.1, Addendum, first.

DOI: 10.1201/9781003527749-12

12.2 THE ROLE OF ICTS IN GLOBAL COLLABORATIONS

In an interconnected world, ICTs serve as the backbone of global collaborations. They enable communication, knowledge sharing, and real-time data exchange across borders, which are all essential for collaborative efforts in medical physics. Through platforms like email, video conferencing, cloud computing, and collaborative software, ICTs allow medical physicists, clinicians, and researchers to work together regardless of their geographic locations.

12.2.1 Key ICTs in Global Medical Physics Collaborations

1. **Video Conferencing:** Tools like Zoom, Skype, and Microsoft Teams have revolutionized the way teams communicate and collaborate. These technologies allow real-time, face-to-face discussions, helping to bridge the physical distance between professionals in different countries. Video conferencing is particularly valuable in situations where in-person interactions are not possible due to time or financial constraints.

2. **Cloud Computing:** Platforms such as Google Drive, Dropbox, and specialized medical databases enable the sharing of large datasets, research findings, and even clinical images, which are crucial in medical physics. The cloud provides a secure and accessible means for cross-border sharing of information, making it easier to manage projects, track progress, and collaborate in real time.

3. **Collaborative Software:** Platforms like Slack, Trello, and Microsoft Teams facilitate project management, communication, and workflow management for multidisciplinary teams. These tools streamline collaboration by allowing instant messaging, document sharing, and task delegation across different time zones.

4. **Telemedicine and Teletherapy:** Particularly in low-resource settings, telemedicine platforms offer access to remote consultations and the delivery of medical physics expertise. Teletherapy allows patients in remote or underserved areas to receive radiation treatment consultations and planning services from specialized experts.

12.3 APPLICATIONS OF AI IN GLOBAL COLLABORATIONS

Artificial intelligence is rapidly transforming many fields, including medical physics. AI applications enhance global collaborations by providing advanced tools for data analysis, decision-making, and automation. Medical physics practitioners can leverage AI algorithms to improve diagnostic accuracy, treatment planning, and even predict patient outcomes.

12.3.1 Key Applications of AI in Global Medical Physics Collaborations

1. **Medical Imaging Analysis:** AI-driven image processing tools help in interpreting medical images, such as CT scans, MRIs, and X-rays. Algorithms trained on large datasets are now capable of detecting abnormalities (such as tumours or lesions) with great accuracy. These technologies facilitate collaboration between international teams, as AI models can analyze images remotely and provide standardized diagnostic insights, reducing human error and enhancing decision-making.

2. **Treatment Planning:** AI applications are now used in radiation therapy planning to predict optimal treatment regimens. AI systems can analyze patient data, simulate treatment plans, and optimize radiation doses to ensure the most effective and safe approach. This is especially important in resource-limited settings where medical physicists may lack the expertise to create individualized plans.

3. **Predictive Modelling:** AI algorithms can analyze vast amounts of clinical data to predict patient outcomes, allowing for personalized treatment plans. By identifying trends and making real-time predictions, AI tools help clinicians, medical physicists, and researchers collaborate effectively and anticipate patient needs across different regions.

4. **Automation of Routine Tasks:** AI is also being applied to automate repetitive tasks like quality assurance checks, radiation dose calculations, and equipment calibration, thus freeing up time for professionals to focus on more complex issues. These technologies are particularly useful in busy hospitals where resources are stretched thin.

5. **Machine Learning for Data-Driven Research:** In research settings, AI-driven machine learning algorithms analyze large datasets, assisting in identifying patterns that may not be immediately obvious to human researchers. This ability to manage and extract insights from big data accelerates international collaborations, particularly when researchers from different countries contribute their unique datasets to a shared project.

12.4 MINIMAL REQUIREMENTS FOR SUCCESS IN GLOBAL ICT AND AI APPLICATIONS

While ICTs and AI hold great promise for enhancing global medical physics collaborations, their success is contingent upon several minimal requirements, especially in resource-limited environments. These requirements include:

1. **Reliable Internet Connectivity:** A stable and high-speed internet connection is fundamental for effective use of ICTs and AI in global collaborations. In regions with poor internet infrastructure, technologies may not perform optimally, hindering communication and data sharing.

2. **Data Security and Privacy Protections:** Medical data is sensitive, and ensuring that all ICT and AI platforms comply with international standards for data security (e.g., GDPR, HIPAA) is essential for trust and legal compliance. Collaborations must establish protocols for data handling to protect patient privacy across borders.

3. **Interoperability of Systems:** Different countries and institutions may use different software platforms, data formats, and technologies. Successful global collaboration requires these systems to be interoperable, meaning they can communicate and exchange data seamlessly. Standardization efforts, such as DICOM for medical imaging, help ensure interoperability.

4. **Technical Infrastructure and Training:** Adequate hardware and software infrastructure, including powerful computing systems for AI applications, is necessary to support advanced medical physics tasks. Additionally, training local staff in both high- and low-resource settings to use these technologies effectively is crucial for success.

5. **Cultural Competency:** Given the diverse backgrounds of medical physicists, clinicians, and patients around the world, cultural understanding plays a significant role in the success of ICT and AI collaborations. Teams must be sensitive to cultural differences in communication, expectations, and healthcare delivery.

12.5 BARRIERS AND LIMITATIONS OF ICTS AND AI IN THE GLOBAL CONTEXT

Despite the many advantages, there are significant barriers and limitations to the use of ICTs and AI in global collaborations, particularly in low-income settings.

1. **Infrastructure Gaps:** In low-income countries, access to reliable electricity, high-speed internet, and modern computing hardware remains a critical barrier to the implementation of ICTs and AI technologies. Inadequate infrastructure hinders the ability of professionals to fully engage in global collaborations.

2. **Cost and Resource Limitations:** Advanced AI applications, such as deep learning algorithms, often require significant computational power and expensive hardware. In many low-resource settings, the cost of acquiring such technology is prohibitive. Moreover, ongoing costs related to maintenance, updates, and training can be a significant burden.

3. **Ethical Concerns:** The use of AI raises ethical questions about transparency, accountability, and the potential for bias. In medical physics, AI algorithms that are trained on datasets from high-income countries may not perform well when applied to diverse populations with different demographic characteristics. Ensuring that AI tools are equitable and unbiased across different regions is an ongoing challenge.

4. **Language and Communication Barriers:** While ICTs facilitate global collaboration, language differences can still create misunderstandings or delays in communication. In collaborative teams, especially those with members from different linguistic backgrounds, there is a need for translation tools or multilingual support to ensure effective communication.

5. **Regulatory and Legal Differences:** Each country may have different regulations regarding the use of medical technologies, including ICTs and AI. These regulatory differences can pose challenges when trying to implement cross-border collaborations, particularly with regard to patient data sharing and the approval of AI systems for clinical use.

12.6 SUMMARY

In this chapter, we explored the role of information and communication technologies (ICTs) and artificial intelligence (AI) in global collaborations in the field of medical physics. ICTs have revolutionized the way professionals collaborate internationally, facilitating communication, data sharing, and the execution of joint research projects. Meanwhile, AI applications in medical imaging, treatment planning, and predictive modelling hold great potential for advancing global health initiatives.

However, for these technologies to succeed in global settings, several requirements must be met, including reliable internet connectivity, data security, and cultural competency. Barriers such as infrastructure gaps, cost limitations, and ethical concerns must also be addressed to ensure the equitable use of ICTs and AI across diverse settings.

12.7 RECOMMENDATIONS

1. **Invest in ICT Infrastructure:** Governments and international organizations should prioritize improving internet access and technology infrastructure in low-income countries to support the use of ICTs and AI.

2. **Promote Standardization:** Efforts should be made to standardize data formats and software tools to facilitate seamless communication and data sharing between institutions in different countries.

3. **Ensure Equity in AI Development:** AI models should be trained on diverse datasets to reduce biases and ensure that AI tools are effective for populations from different regions and backgrounds.

4. **Provide Training and Support:** Professional development programmes should be created to train medical physicists and healthcare workers on the use of ICTs and AI, with a focus on ensuring that these tools are accessible to those in low-resource settings.

5. **Encourage Multilingual Communication:** Tools for real-time translation and multilingual support should be incorporated into ICT platforms to overcome language barriers in global collaborations.

6. **Strengthen Data Privacy and Security:** International standards for data privacy should be adhered to, and collaboration agreements should include robust measures to protect patient information.

12.A.1 ADDENDUM

Sections 12.1–12.7 were written by the free version of ChatGPT-4o mini. On 22 January 2025, it was given the following instructions:

Write a chapter of less than 2500 words with the following considerations:

Book Title: Global Medical Physics: A Guide for International Collaboration.

*The **main purpose** of this book is to provide guidance, primarily to medical physicists, in both low- and high-income countries on issues related to partnering with colleagues in different country settings, especially in the clinical and educational medical physics circles, and also in research and academic environments. There is also a growing interest in short-term experiences in global health (STEGHs). However, in some cases, these STEGHs can be counterproductive and even harmful. Furthermore, international engagements may be obstructed by multiple barriers, ranging from cultural, to language, to ethical, to internet and technology limitations.*

The book is intended to be a great resource for undergraduate students, graduate students, and residents wishing to study abroad. Furthermore, it will be a useful guide for anyone wishing to relocate to another country or being involved in short-term experiences in global health.

Chapter number 12.

Chapter title: The Role of Information Computer Technologies (ICTs) and Artificial Intelligence (AI) in Global Collaborations
Chapter sections are numbered as 12.1, 12.2, etc.
Section 12.1 contains the chapter objectives as follows:

- *To describe the use of ICTs for global collaborations*

- *To describe the applications of AI in global collaborations*

- *To suggest minimal requirements for success in global ICT and AI applications*

- *To discuss applications, barriers, and limitations of ICTs and AI in the global context*

- *To provide recommendations regarding the use of ICTs and AI for enhancing global applications*

The last section of each chapter contains two subsections entitled summary and recommendations. The recommendations are listed in point form.

Include citations as appropriate.

No more than three figures.

12.A.2 CRITIQUE

At first glance, this appears to be a reasonably well-written overview regarding ICTs and AI. However, the following are some critiques from which we may be able to learn some lessons.

1. **Overly General**: While the general concepts and issues were addressed, there were few specifics regarding the topics listed. For example, in this book, Chapters 4, 8, 11, 13, and 14 included comments/discussions regarding ICTs and AI. The broad concepts introduced in Chapters 4 and 13 are alluded to in the above write-up, but there were no specifics.

2. **No Citations**: While there was a specific request to include citations, none were provided. For example, there are multiple citations referring to the work of Chapter 4 describing automated treatment planning, only three of which are listed here [1–3]. Other examples of relevant topics and references that could have been addressed include:

   a. Oncology education in Africa [4].

   b. Radiation oncology education [5, 6].

   c. ICTs and AI for radiation oncology [7–11].

   d. The use of large language models in radiation oncology physics [12].

   e. Machine and deep learning in oncology, medical physics, and radiology [13].

f. The use of language generative AI for development and bench-marking radiation therapy teaching support tools [14].

g. The use of ChatGPT in radiology [15, 16].

h. Benefit versus risk of the use of AI for submission of medical physics manuscripts [17].

i. Encouragement for medical physicists to integrate AI in health-care [18].

12.A.3 ADDITIONAL COMMENTS

1. The use of ICTs and AI in healthcare is evolving rapidly, as indicated by the PubMed publications, which have increased by a factor of 20 from 285 in 2010 to 5528 in 2024 (using a search on "information computer technologies and artificial intelligence").

2. As indicated above, the range of applications is very broad ranging from benchmarking examinations to automating procedures such as radiation therapy treatment planning and providing support for diagnostic imaging.

3. ICTs and AI provide tremendous opportunities for improving efficiency and accuracy and levelling the playing field for high-income countries (HICs) and low- to middle-income countries (LMICs).

12.A.4 FURTHER RECOMMENDATIONS FROM CHATGPT

The following is the response from ChatGPT-4o after requesting "Recommendations for Medical Physicists on using ICTs and AI" requested on 28 February 2025.

To quote:

Here are some recommendations for medical physicists on using information and communication technologies (ICTs) and artificial intelligence (AI) in their practice:

1. **Enhance Clinical Practice with AI and ICTs**

- Utilize AI-powered image analysis tools for improved accuracy in medical imaging (e.g., segmentation, anomaly detection).

- Implement ICTs for remote quality assurance, dosimetry verification, and treatment planning.

- Adopt telemedicine platforms for remote consultations and second opinions.

2. Leverage AI for Research and Development

- Use AI models for data analysis in radiotherapy, diagnostic radiology, and nuclear medicine.

- Explore machine learning techniques to optimize radiation therapy planning and predictive modelling.

- Engage in collaborative AI research to improve personalized treatment approaches.

3. Improve Education and Training with Digital Tools

- Incorporate AI-driven simulations and virtual reality (VR) for training in radiation therapy and imaging.

- Utilize online learning platforms, webinars, and massive open online courses (MOOCs) for continuous professional development.

- Encourage the use of AI-assisted tutoring systems for medical physics education.

4. Implement ICTs for International Collaboration

- Use cloud-based platforms for sharing imaging datasets and treatment plans with global teams.

- Participate in international AI-based initiatives for harmonized protocols in medical physics.

- Leverage collaborative software for joint research, training, and project management.

5. Address Ethical and Regulatory Considerations

- Ensure compliance with patient's data privacy laws (e.g., GDPR, HIPAA) when using AI and ICTs.

- Be aware of biases in AI models and work towards fair and transparent AI implementations.

- Stay updated on regulatory guidelines for AI in healthcare and medical physics applications.

6. **Stay Up to Date with Emerging Technologies**

- Engage in AI and ICT training programmes tailored for health-care professionals.

- Attend international conferences and workshops on AI applications in medical physics.

- Collaborate with AI experts and data scientists to integrate AI effectively into clinical workflows.

REFERENCES

1. Netherton, T.J., *et al.*, The Emergence of Artificial Intelligence within Radiation Oncology Treatment Planning. *Oncology*, 2021. **99**(2): p. 124–134.
2. Baroudi, H., *et al.*, Automated Contouring and Planning in Radiation Therapy: What Is 'Clinically Acceptable'? *Diagnostics (Basel)*, 2023. **13**(4).
3. Court, L., *et al.*, Addressing the Global Expertise Gap in Radiation Oncology: The Radiation Planning Assistant. *JCO Glob Oncol*, 2023. **9**: p. e2200431.
4. Asana, L., *et al.*, Using Advanced Information and Communication Technologies to Advance Oncology Education in Africa. *Ecancermedicalscience*, 2021. **15**: p. 1211.
5. Ngwa, W., *et al.*, Closing the Cancer Divide through Ubuntu: Information and Communication Technology-Powered Models for Global Radiation Oncology. *Int J Radiat Oncol Biol Phys*, 2016. **94**(3): p. 440–449.
6. Chow, J.C.L. and K. Li, Developing Effective Frameworks for Large Language Model-Based Medical Chatbots: Insights from Radiotherapy Education with ChatGPT. *JMIR Cancer*, 2025. **11**: p. e66633.
7. Chow, J.C.L., Internet-based computer technology on radiotherapy. *Rep Pract Oncol Radiother*, 2017. **22**(6): p. 455–462.
8. Landry, G., C. Kurz, and A. Traverso, The Role of Artificial Intelligence in Radiotherapy Clinical Practice. *BJR Open*, 2023. **5**(1): p. 20230030.
9. Liu, J., *et al.*, An Overview of Artificial Intelligence in Medical Physics and Radiation Oncology. *J Natl Cancer Cent*, 2023. **3**(3): p. 211–221.
10. Ngwa, W. and T. Ngoma, *Emerging Models for Global Health in Radiation Oncology*. 2016, Bristol, UK: IOP Publishing.
11. Ngwa, W., *et al.*, Potential for information and communication technologies to catalyze global collaborations in radiation oncology. *Int J Radiat Oncol Biol Phys*, 2015. **91**(2): p. 444–447.
12. Holmes, J., *et al.*, Evaluating large language models on a highly-specialized topic, radiation oncology physics. *Front Oncol*, 2023. **13**: p. 1219326.
13. El Naqa, I.M. and M.J. Murphy (Editors), *Machine and Deep Learning in Oncology, Medical Physics and Radiology*. 2022, Switzerland: Springer.

14. Kadoya, N., *et al.*, Assessing knowledge about medical physics in language-generative AI with large language model: using the medical physicist exam. *Radiol Phys Technol*, 2024. **17**(4): p. 929–937.
15. Keshavarz, P., *et al.*, ChatGPT in radiology: A systematic review of performance, pitfalls, and future perspectives. *Diagn Interv Imaging*, 2024. **105**(7–8): p. 251–265.
16. Soleimani, M., *et al.*, Practical Evaluation of ChatGPT Performance for Radiology Report Generation. *Acad Radiol*, 2024. **31**(12): p. 4823–4832.
17. Low, D.A., P.H. Halvorsen, and S.G. Hedrick, Will Large Language Model AI (ChatGPT) Be a Benefit or a Risk to Quality for Submission of Medical Physics Manuscripts? *Med Phys*, 2025. **52**(4): 1974–1977.
18. Wu, D.H., *et al.*, Embracing Real AI: A Call to Action for Medical Physicists in Healthcare. *J Appl Clin Med Phys*, 2024. **25**(9): p. e14456.

CHAPTER 13

Global Collaboration on Data Sharing

K. Ruwani M. Fernando, Dipesh Niraula, Denis Dudas, Andre Dekker, and Issam El Naqa

13.1 CHAPTER OBJECTIVES

- To highlight the need for data sharing in medical physics
- To describe the common data types used in medical physics
- To describe technologies for data sharing (centralized versus distributed)
- To present sample applications of data sharing

13.2 DATA SHARING IN MEDICAL PHYSICS

13.2.1 Need

J.F. Williamson *et al.* in their Medical Physics Dataset Article announcement stated that

> Making this service available to *Medical Physics* authors and readers recognizes that our field is dependent on experimental or computational datasets which are too expensive and difficult to reproduce in the laboratory of every researcher who needs such data. Using the same reference dataset also enables meaningful comparisons [1].

DOI: 10.1201/9781003527749-13

This announcement reflects the tremendous need to have mechanisms to tabulate and exchange information not only related to research but also safety requirements. For instance, the International Atomic Energy Agency (IAEA) has established, SAFRON, Safety in Radiation Oncology, as an integrated reporting and learning system for radiotherapy and radionuclide therapy incidents and near misses.

On the research side, the rise of artificial intelligence (AI) in radiological science, whether diagnostic or therapeutic, and its application has created an additional need for data sharing. AI is a data-driven technology, and having a large amount of representative data is key to its success, whether for diagnostic purposes or therapeutic planning, quality assurance, or outcome predictions [2].

13.2.2 Challenges

In the areas of data science, it has been reported that scientists spend more than 80% of their time on data extraction, data integration, and data cleaning before building AI models. In many applications, data may not be readily available for usage and it needs to be extracted from structured and unstructured data sources, which would require financial and human resources. This becomes more challenging when attempting to aggregate data across multiple institutions. There are regulatory and ethical concerns regarding privacy protection and sharing of patient data that would need to be addressed on top of the technical aspects mentioned earlier [3, 4]. Moreover, institutions are recognizing the value of such data and there seem to be political and/or monetary obstacles as well [5].

13.2.3 Requirements

As noted earlier, data aggregation in traditional centralized databases has been marred with ethical, political, legal, and technical challenges. Therefore, alternatives based on distributed or federated learning, as discussed here, are considered. In either case, to make them usable, an additional step of data harmonization is required as well. The main requirements for data sharing are summarized in Table 13.1.

13.3 DATA TYPES IN MEDICAL PHYSICS

13.3.1 Clinical

Patient demographics and clinical details are the first data collected and generally considered for most medical AI. These may include age, gender,

TABLE 13.1 Requirements for Data Sharing

Requirements	Remarks
Traditional Data Sharing; Centralized Data	
Legal	Submit formal data request application; obtain Institutional Review Board (IRB) approval and sign in a Data-Sharing Agreement.
Security	Store data safely, preferably inside an institutional firewall.
Patient protection	De-identify data to remove Protected Health Information (PHI). Additional preventive steps such as converting dates into time periods are highly encouraged.
Transparency	In all related publications, provide proper acknowledgement to the data source.
Deletion	When the data-sharing period has expired, delete all the data permanently.
Federated Learning; Decentralized Data	
Legal	Draw a Data-Sharing Agreement and seek IRB approval before signing the agreement; SMART IRB (single IRB multiple site) and forming a consortium can alleviate challenges associated with multi-site research.
Security	Conduct architectural review from cyber-security/IT experts to vet the hardware, software, and especially firewall ports that will be utilized in the project.
Technology	*Hardware*: Allocate necessary CPU, GPU, and memory either on-premise or on-cloud (e.g., AWS, Azure). *FL Software*: Install FL software (e.g., NVFlare, Tensor-Flow Federated). *Connectivity*: Monitor connection between FL Server and FL Client and set inbound rules for extra protection (e.g., only allow connection between IP addresses of involved parties).
Data aggregation	Provide data dictionaries to all parties for data aggregation and data wrangling; upload data in data management systems (e.g., XNAT, FlyWheel), which have multiple advantages such as data protection, automation, visualization.
Patient protection	Ask all the participating groups to de-identify data and encourage them to take additional preventive measures.
Transparency	In all related publications, provide proper acknowledgement to the data source.

ethnicity, disease status, comorbidities, and physiological details (e.g., cardiac function tests, pulmonary function tests, body mass index), lab measurements, and histology, as well as socioeconomic factors and other social determinants of health. These data can be structured (i.e., discrete elements in a database), unstructured (e.g., radiology reports and clinical notes), and may need to be abstracted manually or using AI technologies like natural language processing (NLP).

13.3.2 Imaging

Imaging data is perhaps the most prevalent resource for information in radiological sciences. For instance, it is used for disease diagnosis in radiology and for treatment planning in radiotherapy. There are multiple imaging modalities. The most common are radiographs, CT, MRI, ultrasound, PET, and SPECT. They use different imaging principles and provide different information. Diagnostic modalities, such as CT, are usually used for diagnosis and radiotherapy treatment planning. It shows patient anatomy and is used to extract electron densities in the patient's body, which is crucial for subsequent dose calculation. On the other hand, MRI and nuclear medicine modalities (PET and SPECT) can be characterized as not only anatomical but also biological, molecular, or functional imaging. For example, MRI can be employed to quantify tumour proliferation or necrosis, while PET is more suitable for tumour metabolism assessment or the overall cancer staging. The advantage of combining data from more modalities gave rise to PET/CT, which is nowadays commonly used for multiple tasks, including diagnosis, planning, and post-treatment follow-ups.

Techniques involving the extraction of a large number of features from imaging data, quantitative analysis, and relating this to treatment outcomes (clinical endpoints) are called *radiomics*. There are two basic approaches – feature-based (conventional radiomics) and featureless-based (deep learning radiomics) [6]. Feature-based methods utilize hand-crafted features such as shape and texture, which are analytically predefined and capture characteristics and patterns in the analyzed data. Featureless radiomics benefit mainly from advances in the deep learning area, as it works with features that are learned and extracted by neural networks directly.

13.3.3 Molecular Markers

The growth of the fields of biotechnology and bioinformatics has offered numerous valuable tools and data, which can positively contribute towards the accuracy of diagnosis and/or patient-specific models, their clinical translation, and precision medicine in general. A wide range of molecular biomarkers can currently be analyzed. Most commonly, they are obtained by analysis of the tumour genome (genomics), its further transcriptions into RNA (transcriptomics), translations into proteins (proteomics), and finally metabolites (metabolomics). Combining all these biomarkers in patient-specific models is often referred to as a multiomic approach due to the combination of different -omic datasets. Furthermore, extending the multiomics approach by radiomics led to the emergence of radiogenomics as a newer field in radiological sciences [7].

13.3.4 Treatment

Another important type of data involves treatment details from radio-therapy, chemotherapy, immunotherapy, or others. Among these, the most complex and frequently analyzed data in medical physics is radio-therapy treatment planning data. This includes imaging data, delineation of targets and organs at risk (OARs), technical details of the radiation delivery plan, and the final 3D dose distribution within the patient's body. The 3D dose distribution often serves as a valuable source of information, as it is directly linked to tumour local control [8], radiation-induced toxicities in OARs [9], and even overall survival [10]. Traditional clinical metrics derived from the dose distribution are typically associated with dose–volume metrics (i.e., histogram-based features) within a specified OAR or target – common examples include minimum/maximum dose (D_{min}/D_{max}), mean dose (D_{mean}), minimum dose delivered to $X\%$ of the volume (D_X), or the volume receiving at least X Gy (V_X). More advanced metrics, reflecting the biological response of normal tissues and tumours to radiation, are, for example, equivalent uniform dose (EUD) or effective volume (V_{eff}). EUD represents a uniform dose delivered to the volume that yields equivalent outcomes to the actual 3D dose distribution. V_{eff} refers to a hypothetical portion of the target volume that, if receiving the prescription dose while the remaining volume receives 0 Gy, would result in outcomes equivalent to the real dose distribution. However, these traditional metrics have several limitations, particularly considering their inability to capture the spatial relationships of the dose within OARs and target volumes. This restricts their potential for personalized treatment. Therefore, methods are increasingly employed to extract and analyze more sophisticated features, often integrating these with radiomics and other omics data [11].

13.4 TECHNOLOGIES TO FACILITATE IN DATA SHARING

13.4.1 Security Challenges

A set of data protection laws such as the United States' HIPAA Act [12], Canada's PIPED Act [13], the European Union's GDPR [14], China's PIP law [15], Singapore's PDP Act [16], South Korea's PIP Act [17], India's IT Rules [18], Malaysia's PDP Act [19], Australia's MHR Act [20], South Africa's POPI Act [21], Nigeria's DP regulation [22], Kenya's DP Act [23], Ghana's DP Act [24], Argentina's PDP Act [25], and Brazil's LGPD law [26], among many others, mandate utmost care when handling patient data. Although to adhere to the law, institutions have globally placed some form of firewall against cyberattacks, the frequency and sophistication of cyberattacks (e.g., ransomware [27]) for breaching medical records have grown considerably [28]. Such incidents have increased the data security challenges and, in turn, the waiting time required to get approval for new research projects that involve data sharing.

13.4.2 Centralized Databases

There have been several successful applications of centralized databases such as those for radiotherapy safety (e.g., SAFRON, ROSIS [29], and RO-ILS). These tend to be technically easy to maintain (text-based SQL schema) and don't expose patient's private information. Other centralized examples include databases such as The Cancer Imaging Archive (TCIA) [30] and the Medical Imaging and Data Resource Center (MIDRC) [31] sponsored by the US National Institutes of Health (NIH), which require a more intensive structure and maintenance. Centralized databases generally hold large amounts and a variety of data and thus require continuous and extensive resources to maintain. However, this associated operational cost is often justified with the argument that they promote equality among researchers by providing open access to a wealth of data for developing and benchmarking medical AI algorithms.

13.4.3 Federated Learning

Federated learning (FL) [32] is a distributed machine learning (ML) framework that allows the training of models remotely using data from multiple devices or institutions while preserving data privacy. Contrary to traditional centralized training, where all data is collected on a single server, FL enables collaborative training of a shared global model using decentralized data. A typical FL training process involves local model training on client devices, aggregation of updates from local models [33] by a central server, and the redistribution of the updated global model to the client devices. This process is repeated until the global model reaches convergence.

The key features in FL include data decentralization and privacy preservation. As only the model updates, such as model weights, are shared with the central server, while data remains distributed over the clients, this approach facilitates training machine learning models with reduced data privacy risks. Previous studies have proposed incorporating additional privacy-preserving measures [34] such as differential privacy [35], secure multiparty computation [36], or homomorphic encryption [37] to further enhance data privacy. Among the other characteristics of FL are collaborative learning and model personalization. Collaborative learning in an FL setting enhances the model's generalizability and facilitates training in a robust global model as diverse data sources are used to construct the model. Furthermore, by fine-tuning the global model, client devices can produce personalized local models that align with their specific data distributions.

FL has several real-world applications [38–40]. Its properties, such as data decentralization, make it particularly well-suited for privacy-sensitive domains such as healthcare. Nevertheless, the efficacy of FL systems is limited by unique challenges related to heterogeneity, privacy, and scalability [41]. Heterogeneity can arise from variations in patient characteristics (e.g., inter-patient or sub-population heterogeneity), treatment device specification (e.g., site effect), and measurement (e.g., batch and/or site effect). However, it should be noted that many of these heterogeneity challenges also occur in centralized databases if the data stems from different real-world data sources, such as routine cancer care.

While FL reduces the privacy risks as the raw data is not shared, it is still vulnerable to threats like model inversion and adversarial attacks, which could expose sensitive information [42]. Although strategies such as differential privacy or homomorphic encryption have demonstrated some efficacy in enhancing data privacy, they may reduce accuracy or increase computational costs. Another practical challenge in FL is scalability, as effective communication between the devices and server can be complex in FL systems typically comprised of many clients.

13.5 DATA-SHARING EXAMPLES

13.5.1 Centralized Database: SAFRON

The Safety in Radiation Oncology (SAFRON) database is an integrated voluntary reporting system of radiotherapy incidents and near misses. It was established by the IAEA in December 2012. Since its inauguration,

SAFRON has 50 participating medical institutions and hospitals around the world. The system has records of 1300 incident reports covering various types of incidents, including errors and near misses [43]. There are similar continental incident-sharing databases, such as the Radiation Oncology Safety Information System (ROSIS) [29] in Europe and the Radiation Oncology Incident Learning System (RO-ILS) in North America.

13.5.2 Centralized Database: MEDomics

MEDomics is an international consortium that is aimed at creating a secure, dynamic, continuously learning, and expandable infrastructure, designed to constantly capture multimodal electronic health information, including imaging, across a large and multicentric healthcare system. The effort was started by the Medical Physics group at the University of California, San Francisco (UCSF), and it currently includes collaborators at McGill University, Université de Sherbrooke in QC, Canada, OncoRay in Dresden, Germany, and Maastricht University in the Netherlands [44].

13.5.3 Federated Database: euroCAT

The Maastricht Radiation Oncology group established an infrastructure for federated (distributed) learning for privacy-preserving, multicentric, rapid learning healthcare called euroCAT [45]. As a global expansion of this effort, the group collaborated with the University of Michigan and other institutions on federated learning of lung cancer analysis in patients receiving radiotherapy [46]. The infrastructure was developed via a commercial platform known as the Varian Learning Portal (VLP). VLP used a hub and spokes model, where model application and validation are exchanged between a central hub and the institutions. It supported the application of predictive models across multiple institutions with secure communication and no sharing of the data among participants. Data were placed in a triplestore in a subject–predicate–object manner using Radiation Oncology Ontology (ROO). In each institution, data were extracted from the local sources, de-identified, and then mapped to codes and stored in the local triplestore using ROO, which allowed semantic interoperability, i.e., data can be accessed by the ML algorithm using the same query. The coded data were stored in a PostgreSQL database before conversion to triples using the D2RQ platform [47], and then were stored in a Sesame server triplestore. Each institution had its own triplestore, which was queried using SPARQL for AI applications [46]. This federated learning approach is now open-source [48] and actively used in radiother-apy use cases such as rare anal cancer [49].

13.6 SUMMARY AND RECOMMENDATIONS

13.6.1 Summary

Data sharing is a key component of medical physics clinical practice and scientific research. It can be claimed that modern medical physics in its varying disciplines relies on data, and this cannot be truer than in the area of artificial intelligence and personalized medicine.

13.6.2 Recommendations

The following recommendations are compiled based on the summarized requirements in Table 13.1 and learned from the successful examples presented in this chapter (Table 13.2).

TABLE 13.2   Recommendation for Data Sharing.

	Recommendation	Description
1	Clear definition of the goals for data sharing	Establish the specific objectives of data sharing, whether for radiation safety studies or for AI predictive analytics.
2	Design and develop appropriate infrastructure	This applies to both centralized and decentralized systems. Ensure the necessary software, hardware, and security requirements are in place.
3	Seek willing partners	Form a coalition of willing partners, as it will entail tedious data-sharing agreements and legal documentation.
4	Define data elements to be shared	This is a critical step and is application dependent. Seek the minimum necessary elements to accelerate the process.
5	Apply appropriate data pre-processing	Aggregated data may follow different distributions, and it is important for AI applications, for instance, that the raw data is harmonized.
6	Apply data FAIR (Findable, Accessible, Interoperable, Reusable) principles [50] in your design	Follow these guidelines to organize data so it is easier to find, access, use, and reuse.
7	Share credit	Acknowledge data contributors appropriately to recognize their contributions.

REFERENCES

1. Jeffrey F. Williamson, Shiva K. Das, Mitchell S. Goodsitt, and Joseph O. Deasy. Introducing the medical physics dataset article. *Medical Physics*, 44(2):349–350, 2017.
2. Issam El Naqa, Masoom A Haider, Maryellen L Giger, and Randall K Ten Haken. Artificial intelligence: reshaping the practice of radiological sciences in the 21st century. *British Journal of Radiology*, 93(1106):20190855, 01 2020.
3. Katherine Drabiak, Skylar Kyzer, Valerie Nemov, and Issam El Naqa. AI and machine learning ethics, law, diversity, and global impact. *British Journal of Radiology*, 96(1150):20220934, 05 2023.
4. Dipesh Niraula, Sunan Cui, Julia Pakela, Lise Wei, Yi Luo, Randall K Ten Haken, and Issam El Naqa. Current status and future developments in predicting outcomes in radiation oncology. *British Journal of Radiology*, 95(1139):20220239, 07 2022.
5. Majumder, Mary Anderlik, and Christi J. Guerrini. "Federal privacy protections: ethical foundations, sources of confusion in clinical medicine, and controversies in biomedical research." *AMA Journal of Ethics* 18(3)::288–298, 2016.
6. Michele Avanzo, Lise Wei, Joseph Stancanello, Martin VallŒieres, Arvind Rao, Olivier Morin, Sarah A. Mattonen, and Issam El Naqa. Machine and deep learning methods for radiomics. *Medical Physics*, 47(5):e185–e202, 2020.
7. James T. T. Coates, Giacomo Pirovano, and Issam El Naqa. Radiomic and radiogenomic modeling for radiotherapy: strategies, pitfalls, and challenges. *Journal of Medical Imaging*, 8(3):031902, 2021.
8. Denis Dudas, Paymen Ghasemi Saghand, Thomas J. Dilling, Bradford A. Perez, Stephen A. Rosenberg, and Issam El Naqa. Deep learning-guided dosimetry for mitigating local failure of patients with non-small cell lung cancer receiving stereotactic body radiation therapy. *International Journal of Radiation Oncology*Biology*Physics*, 119(3):990–1000, 2024.
9. Kimberly M. Creach, Issam El Naqa, Jeffrey D. Bradley, Jeffrey R. Olsen, Parag J. Parikh, Robert E. Drzymala, Charles Bloch, and Clifford G. Robinson. Dosimetric predictors of chest wall pain after lung stereotactic body radiotherapy. *Radiotherapy and Oncology*, 104(1):23–27, 2012.
10. Amy C. Moreno, Bryan Fellman, Brian P. Hobbs, Zhongxing Liao, Daniel R. Gomez, Aileen Chen, Stephen M. Hahn, Joe Y. Chang, and Steven H. Lin. Biologically effective dose in stereotactic body radiotherapy and survival for patients with early-stage NSCLC. *Journal of Thoracic Oncology*, 15(1):101–109, 2020.
11. Sunan Cui, Randall K. Ten Haken, and Issam El Naqa. Integrating multiomics information in deep learning architectures for joint actuarial outcome prediction in non-small cell lung cancer patients after radiation therapy. *International Journal of Radiation Oncology*Biology*Physics*, 110(3):893–904, 2021.

12. U.S. Department of Health and Human Services. The HIPAA privacy rule. https://www.hhs.gov/hipaa/for-professionals/privacy/index.html. 45 CFR Part 160 and Subparts A and E of Part 164; Accessed: 2024-12-23.

13. Office of the Privacy Commissioner of Canada. The personal information protection and electronic documents act (PIPEDA), December 8 2021. Office of the Privacy Commissioner of Canada. https://www.priv.gc.ca/en /privacy-topics/privacy-laws-in-canada/the-personal-information-protec-tion-and-electronic-documents-act-pipeda/; Accessed: 2024-12-23.

14. European Parliament and Council of the European Union. Regulation (EU) 2016/679 of the European Parliament and of the Council. European Parliament and Council of the European Union. Regulation (EU) 2016/679 of the European Parliament and of the Council. https://www.legislation .gov.uk/eur/2016/679/contents#:~:text=Regulation%20(EU)%202016/679,) (Text%20with%20EEA%20relevance)

15. Rogier Creemers and Graham Webster. Translation https://digichina.stan-ford.edu/work/translation-personal-information-protection-law-of-the -peoples-republic-of-china-effective-nov-1-2021/. Published by DigiChina, Stanford University; Accessed: 2024-12-23.

16. Government of Singapore. Personal data protection act 2012. https://sso.agc .gov.sg/Act/PDPA2012, 2012. Revised Edition 2020; Accessed: 2024-12-23.

17. Personal Information Protection Commission, Korea. Notice: PIPC offers guideline on processing publicly available data for ai development and ser-vices. https://pipc.go.kr/eng/user/ltn/new/noticeDetail.do?bbsId= BBSMST R_000000000001&nttId=2331, 2024; Accessed: 2024-12-23.

18. Ministry of Electronics and Information Technology, India. Information technology (intermediary guidelines and digital media ethics code) rules, 2021. https://www.meity.gov.in/content/information-technology-inter-mediary-guidelines-and-digital-media-ethics-code-rules-2021; Accessed: 2024-12-23.

19. Government of Malaysia. Personal data protection act 2010. https://www .pdp.gov.my/ppdpv1/en/akta/pdp-act-2010/, 2010; Accessed: 2024-12-23.

20. Government of Australia. My health records act 2012. https://www.leg-islation.gov.au/C2012A00063/latest/text, 1988. Published by the Federal Register of Legislation, Australia; Accessed: 2024-12-23.

21. Government of South Africa. Protection of personal information act 2013. https://www.gov.za/documents/protection-personal-information-act, 2013; Accessed: 2024-12-23.

22. National Information Technology Development Agency, Nigeria. Nigeria data protection regulation 2019. https://nitda.gov.ng/wp-content/uploads /2020/11/NigeriaDataProtectionRegulation11.pdf, 2019; Accessed: 2024-1223.

23. Government of Kenya. Data protection act 2019. https://www.odpc.go.ke/ data-protection-laws-kenya/, 2019. Published by the Office of the Data Protection Commissioner, Kenya; Accessed: 2024-12-23.

24. Government of Ghana. Data protection act 2012. https://nita.gov.gh/wp -content/uploads/2017/12/Data-Protection-Act-2012-Act-843.pdf, 2012. Published by the National Information Technology Agency, Ghana; Accessed: 2024-12-23.

25. Government of Argentina. Law 25.326: protection of personal data, November 2 2000. https://servicios.infoleg.gob.ar/infolegInternet/anexos /60000-64999/64790/norma.htm; Accessed: 2024-12-23.

26. Government of Brazil. General law for the protection of personal data (lgpd, 2018. https://iapp.org/resources/article/brazilian-data-protection-law-lgpd -english-translation/; Accessed: 2024-12-23.

27. Lars Daniel. 100 million Americans' medical records exposed in massive data breach, 2024. https://www.forbes.com/sites/larsdaniel/2024/10/28/100 -million-americans-medical-records-exposed-in-massive-data-breach/; Accessed: 2024-12-27.

28. CM Alliance. October 2024: Biggest cyber attacks, data breaches, ransomware attacks, https://www.cm-alliance.com/cybersecurity-blog/top -10-biggest-cyber-attacks-of-2024-25-other-attacks-to-know-about 2025; Accessed: 2025-01-20.

29. Cunningham J, Coffey M, Knöös T, Holmberg O. Radiation Oncology Safety Information System (ROSIS): profiles of participants and the first 1074 incident reports. *Radiotherapy & Oncology* 97(3):601–607, 2010 Dec. doi: 10.1016/j.radonc.2010.10.023.

30. Justin Kirby, Fred Prior, Nicholas Petrick, Lubomir Hadjiski, Keyvan Farahani, Karen Drukker, Jayashree Kalpathy-Cramer, Carri Glide-Hurst, and Issam El Naqa. Introduction to special issue on datasets hosted in the cancer imaging archive (TCIA). *Medical Physics*, 47(12):6026–6028, 2020.

31. Naveena Gorre, Eduardo Carranza, Jordan Fuhrman, Hui Li, Ravi K Madduri, Maryellen Giger, and Issam El Naqa. MIDRC CRP10 AI interface—an integrated tool for exploring, testing and visualization of AI models. *Physics in Medicine & Biology*, 68(7):074002, Mar 2023.

32. Brendan McMahan, Eider Moore, Daniel Ramage, Seth Hampson, and Blaise Aguera y Arcas. Communication-efficient learning of deep networks from decentralized data. In *Artificial Intelligence and Statistics*, pp. 1273–1282. PMLR, 2017.

33. Pian Qi, Diletta Chiaro, Antonella Guzzo, Michele Ianni, Giancarlo Fortino, and Francesco Piccialli. Model aggregation techniques in federated learning: a comprehensive survey. *Future Generation Computer Systems*, 150:272–293, 2024.

34. Ziyao Liu, Jiale Guo, Wenzhuo Yang, Jiani Fan, Kwok-Yan Lam, and Jun Zhao. Privacy-preserving aggregation in federated learning: a survey. *IEEE Transactions on Big Data*, 1–20, 2022. doi: 10.1109/TBDATA.2022.3190835.

35. Kang Wei, Jun Li, Ming Ding, Chuan Ma, Howard H Yang, Farhad Farokhi, Shi Jin, Tony QS Quek, and H Vincent Poor. Federated learning with differential privacy: algorithms and performance analysis. *IEEE Transactions on Information Forensics and Security*, 15:3454–3469, 2020.

36. Renuga Kanagavelu, Zengxiang Li, Juniarto Samsudin, Yechao Yang, Feng Yang, Rick Siow Mong Goh, Mervyn Cheah, Praewpiraya Wiwatphonthana, Khajonpong Akkarajitsakul, and Shangguang Wang. Two-phase multiparty computation enabled privacy-preserving federated learning. In *2020 20th IEEE/ACM International Symposium on Cluster, Cloud and Internet Computing (CCGRID)*, pp. 410–419. IEEE, 2020.

37. Haokun Fang and Quan Qian. Privacy preserving machine learning with homomorphic encryption and federated learning. *Future Internet*, 13(4):94, 2021.

38. Li Li, Yuxi Fan, Mike Tse, and Kuo-Yi Lin. A review of applications in federated learning. *Computers & Industrial Engineering*, 149:106854, 2020.

39. Jie Xu, Benjamin S Glicksberg, Chang Su, Peter Walker, Jiang Bian, and Fei Wang. Federated learning for healthcare informatics. *Journal of Healthcare Informatics Research*, 5:1–19, 2021.

40. Tuo Zhang, Lei Gao, Chaoyang He, Mi Zhang, Bhaskar Krishnamachari, and A Salman Avestimehr. Federated learning for the internet of things: Applications, challenges, and opportunities. *IEEE Internet of Things Magazine*, 5(1):24–29, 2022.

41. Tian Li, Anit Kumar Sahu, Ameet Talwalkar, and Virginia Smith. Federated learning: Challenges, methods, and future directions. *IEEE Signal Processing Magazine*, 37(3):50–60, 2020.

42. K. N. Kumar, C. K. Mohan and L. R. Cenkeramaddi, "The Impact of Adversarial Attacks on Federated Learning: A Survey," in IEEE Transactions on Pattern Analysis and Machine Intelligence, 46(5):2672–2691, May 2024, doi: 10.1109/TPAMI.2023.3322785.

43. International Atomic Energy Agency (IAEA). SAFRON reporting and learning system https://www.efomp.org/index.php?r=news/view&id=174 [Accessed: 2025-02-15].

44. Olivier Morin, Martin Vallières, Steve Braunstein, Jorge Barrios Ginart, Taman Upadhaya, Henry C. Woodruff, Alex Zwanenburg, Avishek Chatterjee, Javier E. Villanueva-Meyer, Gilmer Valdes, William Chen, Julian C. Hong, Sue S. Yom, Timothy D. Solberg, Steffen Loïck, Jan Seuntjens, Catherine Park, and Philippe Lambin. An artificial intelligence framework integrating longitudinal electronic health records with real-world data enables continuous pan-cancer prognostication. *Nature Cancer*, 2(7):709–722, 2021.

45. Timo M. Deist, A. Jochems, Johan van Soest, Georgi Nalbantov, Cary Oberije, Seán Walsh, Michael Eble, Paul Bulens, Philippe Coucke, Wim Dries, Andre Dekker, and Philippe Lambin. Infrastructure and distributed learning methodology for privacy-preserving multi-centric rapid learning health care: euroCAT. *Clinical and Translational Radiation Oncology*, 4:24–31, 2017.

46. A. Jochems, T. M. Deist, I. El Naqa, M. Kessler, C. Mayo, J. Reeves, S. Jolly, M. Matuszak, R. Ten Haken, J. van Soest, C. Oberije, C. FaivreFinn, G. Price, D. de Ruysscher, P. Lambin, and A. Dekker. Developing and validating a

survival prediction model for NSCLC patients through distributed learning across 3 countries. *International Journal of Radiation Oncology, Biology, Physics*, 99(2):344-352, 2017.

47. Bizer C, *et al.* D2RQ: Accessing relational databases as virtual RDF graphs, http://d2rq.org/ [Accessed: 2025-02-08]
48. Moncada-Torres A, Martin F, Sieswerda M, Van Soest J, Geleijnse G. VANTAGE6: an open source priVAcy preserviNg federaTed leArninG infrastructurE for Secure Insight eXchange. *AMIA Annual Symposium Proceedings*. 2020:870–877, 2021 Jan 25.
49. Choudhury A, Theophanous S, Lønne PI, Samuel R, Guren MG, Berbee M, Brown P, Lilley J, van Soest J, Dekker A, Gilbert A, Malinen E, Wee L, Appelt AL. Predicting outcomes in anal cancer patients using multi-centre data and distributed learning – A proof-of-concept study. *Radiotherapy & Oncology* 159:183–189, 2021 Jun. doi: 10.1016/j.radonc.2021.03.013.
50. Wilkinson, M., Dumontier, M., Aalbersberg, I. *et al.* The FAIR Guiding Principles for scientific data management and stewardship. *Science Data* 3, 160018, 2016. https://doi.org/10.1038/sdata.2016.18.

CHAPTER 14

Global Collaborations: The European Council for Nuclear Research (CERN) Perspective

Laurence Wroe, Steinar Stapnes, and Manjit Dosanjh

14.1 CHAPTER OBJECTIVES

- To describe CERN's experience with international engagement

- To outline CERN's strategic plan for international collaborations

- To review CERN's experience with implementation of strategic plan for international activities

- To summarize CERN's involvement in enhancing international collaborations for medical physicists

14.2 THE CERN ORGANIZATION AND COLLABORATIVE PROJECTS WITHIN PARTICLE PHYSICS

The European Council for Nuclear Research (CERN) is an intergovernmental organization comprised of 24 Member States. The CERN laboratory is located on the France–Switzerland border close to the city of

DOI: 10.1201/9781003527749-14

Geneva where it hosts a wide range of experiments and facilities, including the Large Hadron Collider (LHC), which is the largest and most powerful particle accelerator in the world. CERN's primary mission is to carry out a diverse research programme at the cutting-edge of fundamental physics research, with education and training, technology development, and international collaboration, each being important as complementing and facilitating parts of the organization's mission.

Global collaboration has been at the heart of CERN's ethos since its founding in 1954 by 12 European countries in the backdrop of the Second World War. CERN was one of Europe's first joint ventures and a forerunner of the 1958 founding of the European Economic Community (EEC). It has since expanded globally to comprise 24 Member States, 2 Associate Member States in the pre-stage to Membership, 8 Associate Member States, 3 countries and 3 international organizations with Observer status, 44 Non-Member States with co-operation agreements, and numerous other countries in scientific collaboration [1]. Around 3,500 staff and associated personnel are engaged by CERN, and it additionally hosts approximately 12,400 visiting scientists and researchers from Universities and Institutes worldwide, with roughly 7,000 people entering the site daily [2].

Throughout its 70-year history, the CERN Convention and Financial Protocol has remained almost unchanged. The Convention contains 20 articles and outlines CERN's spirit to

> provide for collaboration among European States in nuclear research of a pure scientific and fundamental character, and in research essentially related thereto,... with no concern with work for military requirements and the results of its experimental and theoretical work shall be published or otherwise made generally available [3].

Such statements are important reasons why CERN has been so successful in engaging a worldwide community in its programme to investigate fundamental physics questions by exploiting an ever-advancing accelerator complex that collides particles at the highest possible energies and intensities.

Today CERN operates several accelerators on its premises, in many cases linking them together to progressively inject into the larger ones.

CERN naturally takes the lead role in the construction, improvement, and operation of its accelerator complex, although with important contributions often made of in-kind components and parts from key international partners, typically national laboratories with strong accelerator expertise. The experimental facilities that make use of these accelerators, for example LHC detectors, are organized differently as large international collaborations with many partners. For these highly distributed collaborations, CERN is typically a partner at 20% level and provides the all-important host and integration support, but most of the component construction, operation responsibilities, and computing and data analyses are carried out by worldwide collaborations. This allows for a very efficient use of scientific, technological, and industrial expertise in a worldwide network to build unique and very complicated integrated systems. For example, the ATLAS and CMS experiments at the LHC each have close to 200 participating institutions from around 50 countries, and thousands of students from the collaborating institutions are at any given time making use of the data from these experiments for their thesis projects. Such decentralized yet tightly coordinated collaborations serve as good models for technology transfer projects. This includes medical applications, where academic, medical, and industrial experts from collaborating partners outside of CERN benefit from working together with technology experts at CERN, particularly within the domains of accelerators, detectors, and computing, to address specific challenges of novel applications.

14.3 CERN'S EXPERIENCES IN MEDICAL PHYSICS COLLABORATIONS

CERN has a rich history of collaboration in medical physics, with the active involvement of its personnel and technologies tracing back to pioneering efforts in the 1970s. One such example is Georges Charpak whose 1968 invention of the multiwire proportional chamber (MWPC) enabled the detection of thousands of ionizing particles per second, orders of magnitude more than could be detected with previous technologies. The widespread adoption of MWPCs in particle physics laboratories contributed to many milestone discoveries but Charpak also dedicated significant effort to ensure MWPCs were fully exploited in medical imaging. CERN has since improved upon this technology, and micro-pattern gaseous detectors such

TABLE 14.1   A Non-exhaustive List of CERN's Involvement in Medical Application
Projects and Collaborations That Harness Its Detector Expertise

Detector Technology/ Expertise	Collaboration/Project Active Years	Brief Description
Scintillators	Crystal Clear Collaboration (CCC) [5] 1990–ongoing	First established with the aim of developing inorganic scintillators suitable for use in CERN detectors, the CCC also branched out into the development of medical imaging devices. In particular, the CCC developed PET modules with depth of interaction and timing capabilities that have been utilized in a number of PET devices, including the breast imaging scanner, CLEARPEM, and the multimodal imaging technique for endoscopic examination of the pancreas and prostate, EndoTOFPET-US.
Pixel detectors	Medipix [6] 1997–ongoing	The first demonstration of large-area hybrid pixel detectors in a high-energy physics experiment was in CERN's WA97 experiment in 1995. The Medipix1 collaboration spun out from this to develop the first large-area, single-photon-counting CMOS imaging chip with the aim of improving contrast resolution in medical imaging applications. Medipix2, Medipix3, and Medipix4 collaborations have since developed a series of pixel detector read-out chips for particle imaging and detection in a wide range of applications, including the creation of the first human 3D colour X-ray image by MARS Bioimaging using Medipix3.

as gaseous electron multipliers (GEMs) continue to find modern applications in medical diagnostics [4]. An additional example of an early pioneer is David Townsend who started working on positron emission tomography (PET) technologies whilst at CERN in 1975. Townsend continued to collaborate with CERN staff in the 1980s after moving to the Cantonal Hospital in Geneva and he went on to construct the first PET-CT.

Since then, CERN has been involved in many medical collaborations and projects. Tables 14.1–14.3 briefly and non-exhaustively summarize a list of medical-related topics and directions where CERN has been and/or is involved in at a significant level using its expertise in accelerators, detectors, and computing.

TABLE 14.2   A Non-exhaustive List of CERN's Involvement in Medical Application Projects and Collaborations That Harness Its Accelerator Expertise

Accelerator Technology/ Expertise	Collaboration/Project Active Years	Brief Description
Hadron accelerator design	PIMMS (Proton-Ion Medical Machine Study) [7] 1996–2000	Growing interest towards hadron therapy in the 1990s led to the establishment of PIMMS to design a state-of-the-art light-ion hadron therapy facility. The project was carried out under the technical leadership of CERN, whose expertise in hadron accelerator design was particularly necessary for the smooth and controllable delivery of proton and carbon ion beams to the required specification, and in collaboration with TERA, MedAustron, Onkologie 2000, and, initially, GSI. The PIMMS facility design was outlined in two design reports that are freely available and led to the construction of two facilities in Italy and in Austria.
	NIMMS (Next Ion Medical Machine Study) [8] 2019–ongoing	Building on the success of PIMMS, CERN launched NIMMS to develop the next generation of heavy-ion therapy centres. The project is based at CERN and involves nearly 20 international partners who aim to advance technology in four key areas: smaller synchrotrons for particle therapy, curved superconducting magnets for synchrotrons and gantries, superconducting gantry designs, and high-frequency ion linacs.
	BioLEIR [9] 2012–2017	At the 2010 Physics for Health in Europe (PHE) conference, members of the biomedical and physics community asked CERN to lead an initiative that would tackle the need for an open-access biomedical facility dedicated to radiobiological and radiophysical research for optimizing hadron therapy. In response, CERN published a feasibility study for BioLEIR, which would adapt CERN's existing Low Energy Ion Ring (LEIR) such that it could be operated in the stoppage period of CERN's heavy-ion physics programme to deliver high-quality light-ion beams for biological, clinical, and medical physics research.

(Continued)

TABLE 14.2 *(Continued)*

Electron accelerator design	STELLA (Smart Technologies to Extend Lives with Linear Accelerators) [10] 2016–ongoing	At the ICTR-PHE 2014 (International Conference on Translational Research in Radio-Oncology and Physics for Health in Europe) co-organized by CERN and ICTR, the global inequality in access to radiotherapy was highlighted in a presentation by the International Cancer Experts Corps (ICEC). Since then, CERN has been continuously involved in the project STELLA which aims to design an adaptable and upgradable, AI-augmented, robust, high-throughput, and affordable electron-based radiotherapy system.
	Deep Electron Flash Facility (DEFT) [11] 2020–ongoing	VHEE (Very-High Electron Energy) Flash-based radiotherapy appears as a promising and tantalizing technique for treating cancer in fewer treatments and with less toxicity. CERN and the Lausanne University Hospital (CHUV) have collaborated alongside an industrial partner to develop the conceptual design of the DEFT facility which exploits CERN accelerator technology to fit within a hospital campus and budget. CERN also hosts the CLEAR (CERN Linear Electron Accelerator for Research) facility, which is an electron accelerator suitable for undertaking research into the medical applications of electron beams in the Flash and VHEE regimes.
Radioisotope production	ISOLDE (Isotope Separator On Line Device) [12] 1967–ongoing	The ISOLDE facility is part of CERN's experimental facilities and provides radioactive ion beams to users in the fields of nuclear, atomic, molecular, particle, astro-, bio-, and solid-state physics. Sixteen countries comprise the ISOLDE collaboration and its user community involves over 900 people.
	MEDICIS (MEDical Isotopes Collected from ISOLDE) [13] 2010–ongoing	The MEDICIS facility uses radioactive isotopes produced at ISOLDE to support the research and development for using non-conventional radionuclides in nuclear medicine. Theranostics and targeted radionuclide therapy are particular research aims. MEDICIS also supports the PRISMAP (PRoduction of high-purity Isotopes by mass Separation for Medical APplication) European medical radionuclide programme with its goal in providing a sustainable source of high-purity radioisotopes for medicine.

(Continued)

TABLE 14.2 (*Continued*)

Collaboration and network building	ENLIGHT (European Network for Light-Ion Therapy) [14] 2002 –ongoing	ENLIGHT formed to allow collaboration between the physics, oncological, radiobiological, engineering, and computing groups in international academic, research, and industrial settings that were interested in the emergence of light-ion therapy centres. It was one of the first clear examples of exporting CERN's collaborative philosophy into a medical environment and ENLIGHT now involves more than 1,000 participants from 50 European countries. ENLIGHT has acted as an umbrella for coordinating a number of projects including: PARTNER (Particle Training Network for European Radiotherapy); ENVISION to develop novel imaging modalities that provide real-time information and quality assurance on delivered doses; ENTERVISION, a complementary training network with ENVISION; and ULICE (Union of Light-Ion Therapy Centres in Europe), an infrastructure project with 20 institutes and provided international access to hadron beams.
	HITRIplus (Heavy-Ion Therapy Research Integration plus) [15] 2020–ongoing	CERN is a key partner of HITRIplus, a collaboration of 18 institutes that aims to integrate biophysics and medical research on cancer treatment with heavy-ion beams while jointly developing the next generation of instruments. Another key partner is the South East European International Institute for Sustainable Technologies (SEEIIST) which was proposed in 2016 by CERN's former Director General Herwig Schopper. SEEIST's objective is to build a facility for hadron therapy for Southeastern European countries whilst incorporating the spirit of CERN by promoting collaboration to mitigate tensions between countries in the region and to provide educational and training platforms. Taking inspiration from this, another initiative was started in 2021 by the CERN Baltic Group to bring a novel and first hadron therapy centre to the Baltic region.

TABLE 14.3   A Non-exhaustive List of CERN's Involvement in Medical Application Projects and Collaborations That Harness Its Computing Expertise

Computing Technology/ Expertise	Collaboration/Project Active Years	Brief Description
Information sharing	The World Wide Web 1989–1993	Arguably CERN's most important contribution to society is the World Wide Web. Invented to solve the inefficiencies associated with finding information stored on different computers and with information sharing between scientists around the world, the World Wide Web was further developed by CERN, US particle physics laboratories, and universities around the globe until CERN released the World Wide Web source code into the public domain as open-source software.
Collaboration building	CERN openlab [16] 2001–ongoing	The CERN openlab is a unique public–private partnership between CERN and leading ICT companies. Within this framework, CERN provides access to its computing infrastructure and expertise in order to provide a demanding environment in which industry collaborators can test their products. Among many, CERN's openlab birthed the innovative tool BioDynaMo (Biology Dynamics Modeller) that aims to provide the most efficient and high-performance simulation platform for agent-based models in a diverse range of use-cases.
Grid computing	Mammogrid [17] 2002–2005 Health-e-Child [18] 2006–2008	CERN adopted grid computing in 2002 to prepare for the analysis of the huge amount of data that the LHC would produce which was beyond CERN's direct computing, financial, or human resources. The WLCG (Worldwide LHC Computing Grid) is now the world's largest computing grid comprising over 170 computing facilities in a worldwide network across 42 countries.

(Continued)

TABLE 14.3 (*Continued*)

		Grid-computing infrastructure, however, also plays a key role in medical applications and two original projects were initiated by CERN: MammoGrid, a Europe-wide distributed database of mammograms, and Health-e-Child, a grid-based integrated healthcare platform for paediatrics that performs epidemiological studies across Europe.
Algorithms	CAFEIN [19] 2019–ongoing	CERN has used federated learning to enable the local training of AI models at different points on the 27 km circumference LHC to minimize the need for data transfers and central storage whilst enhancing efficiency and reinforcing privacy. Such benefits are also desired by the healthcare sector and CERN's CAFEIN platform demonstrated this in hosting an automatic brain MRI Screening Tool for detecting tumour-like pathologies. Since then, a collaboration between CERN and 11 partners across Europe has formed to carry out the TRUSTroke (Trustworthy AI for Improvement of Stroke Outcomes) project.

14.4 CERN'S STRATEGY FOR COLLABORATION OUTSIDE ITS CORE MISSION, INCLUDING MEDICAL APPLICATIONS

The technologies and methods used for the construction, operation, and development of large research facilities, such as CERN's accelerator, detector, and computing systems, in many cases open for applications and innovations outside fundamental research. Initially, such involvements at CERN resulted from a more passive and spontaneous unplanned spread of new ideas; however, the founding of the Industry and Technology Liaison Office in 1988 allowed CERN to pivot into actively disseminating and transferring its knowledge and technology. Now known as the knowledge transfer (KT) group, its priority is on societal impact rather than revenue return which, in turn, can enhance support for its future accelerator projects. Specifically, the KT mandate is to "maximise the technological and knowledge return to the Member States and promote CERN's image as a centre of excellence for technology," and for this it employs some different strategies: the licensing of intellectual property and technology; service, consultancy, collaboration, and partnerships agreements; open-source software; open hardware; spin-off and start-up companies; EU projects; human capital; and the international collaboration in the medical field [20].

This active pursuit of knowledge transfer allows CERN to positively impact society far beyond the domain of fundamental high-energy physics research and by collaborating with international organizations outside of science and technology, CERN can further such impacts. UN Secretary-General Kofi Annan highlighted the need for such collaboration in his 2003 challenge to the world's scientists to help balance the global distribution of scientific activity and decelerate the ever-increasing disparities between advanced and developing countries [21]. CERN responded to this by hosting the 2003 conference on the Role of Science in the Information Society (RSIS), and its results were presented by then Director General Luciano Maiani at the World Summit on the Information Society (WSIS) to emphasize the commonalities between CERN's and the UN's activities. Such developments seeded the granting of CERN's Observer status to the United Nations General Assembly in 2012 [22].

The guiding framework, organization, and strategy of the Medical Applications group of KT were updated in 2017 [23]. It outlines the alignment between CERN's mission and the application of knowledge transfer activities for the benefit of the medical community, highlighting the need to: focus medical applications-related activities on R&D projects using technologies and infrastructures that are uniquely available at CERN, particularly with regard to accelerators, detectors, and computing; engage and align with the Member State medical research communities; carry out projects with clear deliverables and milestones; ensure external stakeholders provide the necessary funding to deliver their projects.

14.5 SUMMARY AND KEY POINTS

14.5.1 Summary

Collaboration has been at the heart of CERN's ethos since its conception and has been essential for the global particle physics community to pursue and attain its ambitious goals [24]. At a high level, CERN is guided by its Convention that has only been amended once in its 70-year history. The Member States forming the CERN Council enforce and ensure the compliance of proposals with the Convention and, ultimately, the projects and collaborations that CERN forms and that its staff operate within.

Taken all together, this forms the so-called "CERN Model," and many institutes/organizations have been founded drawing inspiration from its principles, including: SESAME (Synchrotron-Light for Experimental Science and Applications in the Middle East), the European Molecular Biology Laboratory, the European Space Agency, the European Southern Observatory, the IPCC (Intergovernmental Panel on Climate Change), the World Weather Watch, and the ISCU (International Council for Science) [25].

14.5.2 Key Points

The CERN Model has achieved great success, and it has been suggested that this is due to four prominent reasons [24]:

- A flat hierarchy that allows ideas to be easily pitched and then judged on their intellectual merit.

- A light managerial and organizational structure that encourages the expression of initiatives, ideas, and creativity of individuals.

- A consensus-led decision-making processes.

- A strong common passion for science.

These salient points are the lifeblood of CERN and its collaborations, and their adoption could be beneficial to enhance international collaboration within the medical physics community.

REFERENCES

1. CERN, "Our Member States", https://home.cern/about/who-we-are/our-governance/member-states. [Accessed 28 November 2024].
2. CERN, "Environment Report 2021–2022", https://e-publishing.cern.ch/index.php/CERN_Environment_Report/issue/view/156/121. [Accessed 28 November 2024].
3. CERN, "Convention for the Establishment of a European Organization for Nuclear Research", https://council.web.cern.ch/index.php/en/content/convention-establishment-european-organization-nuclear-research. [Accessed 28 November 2024].
4. *Gaseous Electron Multiplier*, https://gdd.web.cern.ch/gem/. [Accessed 28 November 2024].
5. *The Crystal Clear Collaboration*, https://crystalclearcollaboration.web.cern.ch/. [Accessed 28 November 2024].
6. *Medipix Collaboration*, https://medipix.web.cern.ch/. [Accessed 28 November 2024].
7. L. Badano, *et al.*, *Proton-Ion Medical Machine Study (PIMMS) 1*. 2000. CERN-PS-99-010-DI. https://cds.cern.ch/record/385378 [Accessed 30 August 2025]
8. M. Vretenar and E. Benedetto, "New Accelerator Designs: NIMMS," *Health Technol.*, vol. 14, no. 5, pp. 945–955, 2024.
9. S. Ghithan, *et al.*, "Feasibility Study for BioLEIR", *CERN Yellow Reports: Monographs*, 2017. CERN-2017-001-M. https://cds.cern.ch/record/2260516 [Accessed 30 August 2025]
10. M. Dosanjh, *et al.*, "Developing Innovative, Robust and Affordable Medical Linear Accelerators for Challenging Environments," *Clin Oncol.*, vol. 31, no. 6, pp. 352–355, 2019.
11. C. Rossi, et al., "The Deep Electron Flash Therapy Facility," *Proc. LINAC2024*, pp. 551–556, 2024.
12. *ISOLDE*, https://home.cern/science/experiments/isolde. [Accessed 28 November 2024].
13. *MEDICIS*, https://home.cern/science/experiments/medicis. [Accessed 28 November 2024].
14. *The European Network for Light Ion Hadron Therapy*, https://enlight.web.cern.ch/enlight. [Accessed 28 November 2024].
15. *Heavy Ion Therapy Research Integration Plus*, https://www.hitriplus.eu/. [Accessed 28 November 2024].
16. R. Warren, *et al.*, "Mammogrid — A Prototype Distributed Mammographic Database for Europe," *Clin Radiol.*, vol. 62, no. 11, pp. 1044–1051, 2007.
17. K. Skaburskas, *et al.*, "Healthe-Child: A Grid Platform for European Paediatrics," *J Phys Conf Ser.*, vol. 119, p. 082011, 2008.
18. *CERN Openlab*, https://openlab.cern/. [Accessed 28 November 2024].

19. *CERN CAFEIN,* https://knowledgetransfer.web.cern.ch/kt-fund/projects /cafein-federated-network-platform-development-and-deployment-ai -based-analysis-and. [Accessed 28 November 2024].

20. V. Nilsen and G. Anelli, "Knowledge Transfer at CERN," *Technol Forecast Social Change.*, vol. 112, pp. 113–120, 2016.

21. K. Annan, "A Challenge to the World's Scientists," *Science.*, vol. 299, no. 5612, pp. 1485–1485, 2003.

22. UN General Assembly, "Observer Status for the European Organization for Nuclear Research in the General Assembly", 2012.

23. CERN, "Strategy and Framework Applicable to Knowledge Transfer by CERN for the Benefit of Medical Applications", 2017.

24. M. Dosanjh, "Collaboration: The Force That Makes the Impossible Possible," *Adv Radiat Oncol.*, vol. 7, p. 100966, 2022.

25. A. Schaeffer, *et al.*, "The CERN Model, United Nations and Global Public Goods: Addressing Global Challenges", 2015. https://cds.cern.ch/ record/2271745/files/Report_TheCERNmodel_theUN_andGlobalPublic-Goods_Final_20.04.2017.pdf [Accessed 30 August 2025].

CHAPTER 15

Ethical Considerations in Global Interactions

Gerald A. White

15.1 CHAPTER OBJECTIVES

- To describe ethical considerations related to global collaborations

- To provide examples of ethical concerns related to global collaborations

- To describe education and training considerations, especially for medical physicists involved in global collaborations

- To provide recommendations regarding ethical concerns in global collaborations

15.2 INTRODUCTION

In setting the stage for a discussion of ethical issues in medical physics–related collaborations among practitioners whose professional (and personal) experiences span possibly different geographic, cultural, and economic landscapes, we may find some comfort in knowing that within the foundations upon which ethical arguments are based, we will find diversity of thought and conclusions. This will, hopefully, relieve us of any self-imposed burden that requires us to follow a single "right" path but rather provide guidance and tools to enable us to choose what may be one of several ethically grounded paths in a particular situation, and assist us

DOI: 10.1201/9781003527749-15

to avoid ethically problematic actions that might result from overly constrained concepts of ethical imperatives.

Let us recognize that there is a tension that may arise in our interactions with others, and in global medical physics collaborations in particular, that may need to be resolved by a consideration of "virtue." In the construct of the Greek philosopher Aristotle, virtue is an attribute that moderates the passions. Every virtue is a mean between vices; an attribute that exists in excess or in deficiency is a vice, and in the mean we find virtue. For example, "With regard to honor and dishonor, the mean is proper pride, the excess is known as a sort of 'empty vanity' and the deficiency is undue humility" [1]. Here we find Aristotle classifying humility as a vice, at least "undue" humility. A somewhat contrary view is offered by Augustine of Hippo (now Annaba, Algeria), elevating humility to a virtue in itself "Humility is the foundation of all the other virtues hence, in the soul in which this virtue does not exist there cannot be any other virtue except in mere appearance" [2].

Let us consider one additional concept that we might find useful in analyzing and responding to the various real-life ethical issues in the medical physics global collaboration field. Mohandas Gandhi calls us to consider the term *Satyagraha* [3], coined in connection with the movement for Indian independence, but useful in our context as well. Created from the Sanskrit words *satya* (truth) and *agraha* (polite insistence), the word offers guidance and support in our interactions in a global collaboration context.

The concepts immediately above have been chosen from a panoply of ethical imperatives and models, not to the exclusion of others but rather to highlight frequently cited pressure points in global collaborations and to emphasize the importance of both adherence to principle and sensitivity to context, often in conflict and in need of resolution.

At a more detailed level, there are ethical considerations that have been promulgated by a variety of professional, regulatory, and non-governmental entities. It is worthwhile to review some that have achieved widespread consensus as to value and need for implementation. The International Council on Radiation Protection (ICRP) has published a list of four core ethical values [4] that, while focused on radiological protection, are relevant to this discussion as we will find them applicable to both patient specific and institutionally broad ethical discussions.

The ICRP notes that these values are shared across geographic and cultural borders and thus will be of interest to anyone engaged in global medical physics collaborations. They are summarized as follows.

- **Beneficence and Non-maleficence:** An elaboration of the missive "do no harm," the principle calls for the intended action to provide benefit to the recipient, while avoiding harm. Although separately stated, achieving beneficence and non-maleficence is typically components of the same decision-making process and resultant action and should be considered together. In the global outreach setting, the "recipient" of an action might be an individual patient, a group of patients, or perhaps a group or institutional entity such as a medical practice, research group, hospital department, etc. Differing cultural, technical, or resource backgrounds of the discussants may lead to differing understandings of the relative beneficence and non-maleficence of actions and must be fully and carefully discussed during the decision-making process.

- **Prudence:** Medical decision-making is oftentimes grounded in a knowledge base that offers less than certainty. Prudence is the value that allows the decision-makers grace to make decisions in which there is an associated uncertainty. In biomedical ethics, there is a "precautionary principle" that when there are uncertainties about the future risks of certain policies or actions, one should refrain from such actions or policies [5]. In some areas of endeavour, prudence would advise adherence to a policy of non-maleficence, perhaps precluding action when the beneficial result might have uncertainty attached. In medical decision-making, this interpretation of prudence is not always strictly applicable. In Publication 138 [4], the ICRP summarizes the applicability of the prudence concept in our context:

  > Prudence is the ability to make informed and carefully considered choices without full knowledge of the scope and consequences of actions. It is also the ability to choose and act on what is in our power to do and not to do.

  In global collaborations, one may find that uncertainties in medical (or research or education) decision-making can be complicated by geographic, cultural, or resource-based perceptions of the participants as to the likelihood of a particular outcome. Prudence then becomes a bit more complicated of a value to follow, but does not diminish in importance.

- **Justice:** Ethical issues described by the value "Justice" in the health-care realm are typically focused on problems associated with a mismatch between needs and resources (Distributive Justice). Such discussions become more frequent and acute in the context of global medical physics collaborations, as such collaborations may well involve connections among partners from a range of income groups [6]. It is worth noting that even within a country or region, there may be a wide variation of resource availability [7], and that recognizing such granularity can be important to collaborations. Basil Varkey offers a clear description of principles of Distributive Justice.

  > These are distribution to each person (i) an equal share, (ii) according to need, (iii) according to effort, (iv) according to contribution, (v) according to merit, and (vi) according to free-market exchanges. Each principle is not exclusive, and can be, and are often combined in application. It is easy to see the difficulty in choosing, balancing, and refining these principles to form a coherent and workable solution to distribute medical resources [8].

  In the context of patient care, most would agree that resource allocations might properly be based on need, likely short- and long-term benefit to the patient, acute versus chronic conditions, perhaps even some randomization protocol, etc. In research activities, patient selection might include eligibility criteria that reflect the design of the study. In both the research and clinical care settings, selection should not be influenced by economic, social, legal status, or political considerations.

- **Dignity:** The Universal Declaration of Human Rights begins, in Article 1: "All human beings are born free and equal in dignity and rights" [9]. Dignity, then, in this context, establishes a status of each person that must be respected and carries with it a corollary of autonomy, often described in the same ethical value heading as dignity. Ethical considerations associated with dignity/autonomy are strongly associated with issues of informed consent, a process that may assume additional complexity in the face of global collaborations where concepts of personal autonomy, the constraint of informed consent, and economic and cultural constraints that may lead to differing understandings of the characteristics of informed consent. Additional guidance in this regard (and with respect to the other values listed in this section) may be found in the Belmont Report [10]. This document, while focused on research, also provides relevant guidance with respect to clinical care that might depart from typical practice standards, a situation that may occur when, in a collaboration, practitioners find themselves grounded in differing standards of care. The report is widely recognized as an authoritative resource on biomedical ethics.

15.3 GLOBAL COLLABORATION ACTIVITIES THAT MAY GIVE RISE TO ETHICAL CONSIDERATIONS

In global collaborations, deriving specific pathways of action based upon a limited set of basic values (see above) offers the practitioner the opportunity for enabling creative solutions, but also the opportunity to wander astray. As indicated in the opening paragraphs of this chapter, one may find a variety of pathways forward, but hopefully will find guidance in the basic values enunciated by the ICRP and others referenced earlier. Some specific situations of interest will be found below. They are chosen as examples that may inform interactions, but are not meant to be an exhaustive compilation

15.3.1 Practice Outside of Scope of Training

A frequently reported experience associated with global collaboration programmes is Practice Outside of Scope of Training (POST). There are a number of motivators that may give rise to POST, among them differences in training and practice or differences in specialty descriptions and scope between the visitor and host locations, and, as identified by Doobay-Persaud et al. in a survey of physicians, nurses, nurse practitioners, and physician assistants who were involved in short-term experiences in global health (STEGH) [11]:

- Host expectations not matched with visitor qualifications

- Suboptimal supervision at host sites

- Inadequate preparation to decline a POST request

- Perceived lack of alternatives

- Emergency situations

In her publication, Doobay-Persaud reports informative statistics on the incidences of POST in the survey respondents' STEGH. Informative are three selected quotes from the survey participants. Hopefully, the reader will reflect these responses in the light of the ethical values discussed earlier in this chapter, thus furthering understanding of ethical issues in global collaboration.

> "High-income country (HIC)-trained clinicians often underestimate the capacity and availability of physicians in low-income country (LMIC) settings. They also often fail to completely understand the cultural and structural aspects of the medical systems within these settings." (Resident MD, Obstetrics/Gynaecology)

> "[Visiting clinicians] need to consider urgency of situation and alternatives. Often the person from the HIC is not in the best position to judge this without understanding environment, culture, language. So such decisions should not be taken lightly." (Licensed MD, Family Medicine)

> "For elective cases without imminent danger clinicians should not practice beyond their scope. However, in emergencies, there may be no other alternative. This constitutes a more challenging ethical scenario." (Resident MD, General Surgery)

15.4 RESEARCH CONSIDERATIONS

Research activities in one's home country come with a significant overlay of ethical considerations. Consideration of and compliance with these ethical imperatives require considerable thought, preparation, and execution. Applying ethical principles in situations of global collaboration becomes ever more complex, navigating non-congruent ethical guidelines, identifying ethical guidance that may be universally applicable, and synthesizing mutually acceptable interpretations and implementations of mutually agreed upon general values and principles. Widely accepted national, regional, and international documents will be of help in establishing a mutual foundation for further discussion. Mentioned earlier, global collaboration groups will consider the UN Declaration of Human Rights [9], the Belmont Report [10], and foundational documents such as the Nuremberg Code [12] and the Declaration of Helsinki [13].

Anecdotal reports of ethical considerations in global partnership research abound, many of which will be known to the readers of this chapter from presentations at national and international meetings. Particularly worthy of consideration are issues raised in the recent research by Janina Isabel Steinert *et al.* [14], who report on a systematic review of human subject research in low- and middle-income countries. She identifies several challenges in the conduct of such research that may create ethical conflicts, among them:

- **"Role Conflicts"**: In very low-income settings, staff may be called upon to perform tasks or provide support beyond the scope of the research project. This is analogous to the POST discussion above in clinical practice. Researchers from high-income settings may find ethical conflicts associated with confidentiality, a desire to intervene in cases of extreme medical needs or post-study requests for assistance. Such situations might be anticipated, and ethical guidelines should be constructed *a priori* to provide support for those engaged in the collaboration.

- **"Feelings of Guilt"**: International collaborations between high-income and lower incomes areas are often motivated by a strong sense in the former group participants of contributing to the betterment of the situation of the latter group. This desire, while present in most human research projects, can be exacerbated in global collaboration settings. Clear and mutually agreed upon expectations of the limits of the research project and researcher activities will be useful in mitigating this conflict.

- **"Physical Safety Risks"**: Both local and visiting researchers may find themselves exposed to physical safety risks endemic to the locale, or perhaps exacerbated by a real or perceived sensitivity of the research subject or process. The ethical imperatives of beneficence and non-maleficence described earlier will need to be considered here, with reference to both the study subjects and the research team.

- **"Political Interference"**: All of the values described in the first section of this chapter may need to be invoked with respect to political pressure for a particular design or result of a research study. Research teams may find this pressure applied from within the host locale or from the visiting group home. Also included in this heading would be political repression, travel restrictions, lack of security, or governmental intimidation that might occur in connection with the research study. Both the local and visiting research teams should be aware of the possibility/existence of these potential hazards, keep all team members fully informed, and facilitate discussion on the resolution of these ethical issues.

- **"Inadequate Working Conditions"**: Local and visiting teams may have differing views on the adequacy and justice of working conditions of research staff, particularly local staff. While all participants will want to fully recognize (and candidly discuss) the extent to which cultural and economic differences may suggest ethical concerns to one or the other group, all should recognize that there are well-established ethical norms that should be universally applied [4–10, 12, 13]. Exploitive relationships must be avoided [15].

- **"North-South Power Imbalances"**: Multinational research teams with participants from both HICs and LMICs conducting research in an LMIC country may be reluctant to admit, discuss, or effectively address ethical problems that arise from a history of colonialism or past/continuing economic power imbalances, often connected with racism. Extracting research data and results from low-income countries without compensatory benefits to the country and its residents will certainly raise issues connected with the values of Prudence and Justice. Gauthier Marchais has provided a succinct summary of this topic [16], and with colleagues has published a compelling case study relating unresolved ethical issues and steps forward [17].

- **"Limited Responsiveness of Institutional Review Boards"**: IRBs from either the host or visitor locale may well have differing concepts as to the ethical principles to be applied in a country hosting an international cooperative project. As mentioned above, all should recognize that there are well-established ethical norms that should be universally applied [4–10, 12, 13], yet researchers will also need to take into account local, cultural, economic, and resource conditions.

Global educational partnerships present opportunities that may be less ethically complicated (research subjects and patients may not be involved), but nonetheless require care and caution with the application of ethical principles. Contemporary educators are immersed in an atmosphere of concern for equity, diversity, and inclusion in teaching practices. Tools for honing pedagogic skills in this area are widely available and well publicized, there is no need to reproduce them here. Faculty, whether visiting or remote, may find cultural and resource differences to be more significant than those found in their home classrooms and laboratories, but this is a difference in degree rather than substance. The diverse student population in HICs is a reflection of the mobility of students throughout the world and prepares educators at all levels for work in global collaborations. (The author notes that in the classroom of his grandson in Saskatoon Canada, the most common student birthplace is Saskatchewan, the second most common birthplace is the Democratic Republic of Congo). Curricula will share basic topics common across nations, with modifications as necessary for individual local contexts. The *Open Syllabus Project* of Medical Physics for World Benefit [18] offers a valuable and well-structured opportunity for global collaboration in this regard. Ethical principles in a teaching-focused global collaboration programme will be productively informed by various codes of ethics specific to medical physics that include reference to the education process [19, 20] as well as more general discussions of ethics in teaching [21].

As can be seen from the discussion above, there are common ethical dilemmas in all aspects of global collaboration. Judith Lasker provides a comprehensive and insightful review of ethical processes in short-term global health collaboration activities, analyzing existing guidelines and how they relate to the desires of host communities [22] that will be applicable across all medical physics global collaborations endeavours.

A comprehensive set of recommendations for global health collaborations can be found in the Brocher Declaration [23, 24], some of which are summarized in the recommendations and key points below.

15.5 SUMMARY AND RECOMMENDATIONS/KEY POINTS

15.5.1 Summary

Global collaborations could span different geographic, cultural, and economic landscapes, potentially resulting in circumstances that yield ethical concerns or questions. Some guidance on choices of different ethically grounded paths and assistance for avoiding ethically problematic actions are addressed. The four core ethical values of the International Council on Radiation Protection, which are also relevant to medical physics, are reviewed. These include beneficence and non-maleficence, prudence, justice, and dignity. Some examples are given of global collaboration activities that may give rise to ethical considerations. Ethical issues in the research and teaching contexts are also considered. With application of the ethical principles discussed in this chapter, the participants in global outreach activities will be prepared to identify and respond creatively to ethical challenges encountered in this important work.

15.5.2 Recommendations/Key Points

1. From the Brocher Declaration [23]:

   a. Global health as a field of practice should aim to reduce disparities in health and well-being around the world.

   b. The ethical framework that underlies global engagement is based on principles of mutual respect, solidarity, and social justice.

   c. Communities' needs should be the most critical driver of these activities and should be set by members of the communities themselves in conjunction with the health priorities of the country.

   d. Global health engagements should be sustainable, asset based, bidirectional, adhere to appropriate legal standards, and be adequately evaluated.

2. The following principles should guide all global health engagements [23]:

   a. Mutual partnership with bidirectional input and learning.

   b. Empowered host country and community define needs and activities.

   c. Sustainable programmes and capacity building.

   d. Compliance with applicable laws, ethical standards, and code of conduct.

   e. Humility, cultural sensitivity, and respect for all involved.

   f. Accountability for actions.

3. Take note of and implement the Working Group on Ethics Guidelines for Global Health Training (WEIGHT) [25] developed for institutions, participants, trainees, and sponsors for field-based ethics and best practices.

REFERENCES

1. Aristotle. *Nichomachean Ethics, Book IV*. 350 BCE [Accessed 2024-12-29]; Available from: http://classics.mit.edu/Aristotle/nicomachaen.4.iv.html.
2. Augustine of Hippo. [Accessed 2024-12-30]; Available from: https://elevate-society.com/humility-is-the-foundation-of/.
3. Ghandi, M. [Accessed 2024-12-30]; Available from: https://www.newworl dencyclopedia.org/entry/Satyagraha.
4. ICRP, Ethical foundations of the system of radiological protection. ICRP Publication 138. *Ann ICRP*, 2018. **47**(1).
5. ter Meulen, R.H., The Ethical Basis of the Precautionary Principle in Health Care Decision Making. *Toxicol Appl Pharmacol*, 2005. **207**(2 Suppl): p. 663–667.
6. World Bank. The World by Income and Region. 2024 [Accessed 2024-12-29]; Available from: https://datatopics.worldbank.org/world-development-indicators/the-world-by-income-and-region.html.
7. Lazar, M., S. Thomas, and L. Davenport, Seeking Care at Free Episodic Health Care Clinics in Appalachia. *J Appalach Health*, 2020. **2**(2): p. 67–79.
8. Varkey, B., Principles of Clinical Ethics and Their Application to Practice. *Med Princ Pract*, 2021. **30**(1): p. 17–28.
9. United Nations. Universal Declaration of Human Rights. [Accessed 2024-12-30]; Available from: https://www.un.org/en/about-us/universal-declaration-of-human-rights.
10. National Commission for the Protection of Human Subjects of Biomedical and Behavioral Research. The Belmont Report: Ethical Principles and Guidelines for the Protection of Human Subjects of Research 1979 [Accessed 2024-12-30]; Available from: https://www.hhs.gov/ohrp/sites/default/files/the-belmont-report-508c_FINAL.pdf.
11. Doobay-Persaud, A., *et al.*, Extent, Nature and Consequences of Performing Outside Scope of Training in Global Health. *Global Health*, 2019. **15**(1): p. 60.
12. Weindling, P., The origins of informed consent: the International Scientific Commission on Medical War Crimes, and the Nuremburg code. *Bull Hist Med*, 2001. **75**(1): p. 37–71.
13. World Medical Association. WMA Declaration of Helsinki – Ethical Principles for Medical Research Involving Human Participants. 2024 [Accessed 2024-12-30]; Available from: https://www.wma.net/policies-post/wma-declaration-of-helsinki/.
14. Steinert, J.I., *et al.*, A Systematic Review on Ethical Challenges of 'Field' Research in Low-Income And Middle-Income Countries: Respect, Justice and Beneficence for Research Staff? *BMJ Glob Health*, 2021. **6**(7): e005380.
15. Bangura, I., *et al.*, Ethical Failures in Global Health Research: Violations of Sustainable Development Goal 8, Decent Work for All. *Lancet Glob Health*, 2022. **10**(5): p. e619.

16. Marchais, G. Contemporary Research Must Stop Relying on Racial Inequalities. Africa at LSE 2020 [Accessed 2024-12-30]; 1-8]. Available from: https://eprints.lse.ac.uk/103744/1/Contemporary_research_must _stop_relying_on_racial_inequalities_Africa_at_LSE.pdf.

17. Marchais, G., P. Bazuzi, and A.A. Lameke, 'The Data Is Gold, and We Are the Gold-Diggers': Whiteness, Race And Contemporary Academic Research in Eastern DRC. *Crit African Stud*, 2020. **12**(3): p. 372-394.

18. Medical Physics for World Benefit (MPWB). Open Syllabus Project. 2024 [Accessed 2024-12-30]; Available from: https://mpwb.org/resources/ Documents/OpenSyllabus/output.html.

19. International Atomic Energy Agency (IAEA), *Guidelines on Professional Ethics for Medical Physicists*, TCS 78. 2023, Vienna, Austria: International Atomic Energy Agency (IAEA).

20. Skourou, C., *et al.*, Code of Ethics for the American Association of Physicists in Medicine (Revised): Report of Task Group 109. *Med Phys*, 2019. **46**(4): p. e79–e93.

21. Shapira-Lishchinsky, O., A Multinational Study of Teachers' Codes of Ethics: Attitudes of Educational Leaders. *NASSP Bull.* **104**(1): p. 5–19.

22. Lasker, J.N., *et al.*, Guidelines for Responsible Short-Term Global Health Activities: Developing Common Principles. *Global Health*, 2018. **14**(1): p. 18.

23. Advocacy for Global Health Partnership. The Brocher Declaration. 2020 [Accessed 2024-12-30]; Available from: https://www.ghpartnerships.org/ brocher.

24. Prasad, S., et al., Global Health Partnerships and the Brocher Declaration: Principles for Ethical Short-Term Engagements in Global Health. *Ann Glob Health*, 2022. **88**(1): p. 31.

25. Crump, J.A., J. Sugarman, and Working Group on Ethics Guidelines for Global Health Training, Ethics and Best Practice Guidelines for Training Experiences in Global Health. *Am J Trop Med Hyg*, 2010. **83**(6): p. 1178–1182.

Equity, Diversity, and Inclusion (EDI) in the Global Medical Physics Context

Afua A. Yorke and Iyobosa B. Uwadiae

16.1 CHAPTER OBJECTIVES

- To provide a broad description of Equity, Diversity, and Inclusion (EDI) challenges in the global context

- To describe strategies for promoting EDI in global medical physics including illustrative case histories

- To provide recommendations on addressing EDI issues in the global medical physics context

16.2 EQUITY, DIVERSITY, AND INCLUSION (EDI) IN THE GLOBAL MEDICAL PHYSICS CONTEXT

EDI, these three interconnected concepts, are often discussed together as they are fundamental to creating a fair and inclusive environment. In the context of global medical physics, EDI ensures that every medical physicist, regardless of their geographic location or socioeconomic status, has equal access to opportunities, resources, and recognition within the field.

DOI: 10.1201/9781003527749-16

This is because an internationally diverse and inclusive medical physics community brings together a wide range of perspectives, which can lead to more innovative approaches to solving the complex healthcare challenges that exist across the globe, especially in less-resourced communities.

16.3 HISTORICAL PERSPECTIVE AND CURRENT STATE

EDI in medical physics has been a subject of growing attention globally [1, 2]. Historically, there has been regional dominance in research [3, 4] and technology, underrepresentation of women and minorities, and the uneven distribution of resources and education. Europe and North America have seen a steady rise in technological advancement with modern and sophisticated linear accelerator technologies (conventional linacs, TomoTherapy, Cyber- and Gamma-Knife, Halcyon, MR-Linac, PET-CT-Linac) for radiation therapy, and medical imaging modalities like magnetic resonance imaging (MRI), computed tomography (CT), positron emission tomography (PET), and single-photon emission computed tomography (SPECT). In recent years, there has been a significant increase in contributions to the field from Asia, [5, 6] complementing the traditional dominance of the Western countries. However, there are still significant disparities in the global distribution of research output and access to cutting-edge technologies [7, 8].

In addition to technological advancement, there is the issue of gender balance. Historically, women have been underrepresented in the field of medical physics. Much of the 20th century was predominantly dominated by men, and women were often excluded from key leadership and research roles, which could be attributed to the fact that physics and engineering are entry points into medical physics and these fields have been predominately male dominated [9, 10]. Due to this imbalance, organizations like the American Association of Physicists in Medicine (AAPM) [11–14] and the International Organization for Medical Physics (IOMP) have invested in committee initiatives focused on gender issues and advancement of women in medical physics. Similarly, there are efforts to address the underrepresented racial and ethnic minorities who have in the past been underrepresented in the field. These initiatives have included outreach programmes, scholarships, and mentorship opportunities aimed at increasing diversity within the field.

The impact of colonial legacies has played a huge role in the delay of healthcare infrastructure due to the prioritization of resources for colonial powers [15–17]. This historical inequity has had long-term effects, contributing to the current disparities in medical physics resources and expertise between former colonies and developed nations. These former colonies are often low- to middle-income countries (LMICs) who face significant challenges in accessing modern radiation therapy equipment, medical imaging technologies, and specialized training. As a result, this has led to significant disparities in the quality of cancer care and diagnostic imaging services [18–20] in these regions. The lack of technological advancement has not only left a significant disparity in the care patients receive but has also trickled down to the quality of education they receive, making it difficult for students from LMICs to access the same level of education from their counterparts in the Western countries.

16.4 GLOBAL INITIATIVES FOR EQUITY AND INCLUSION

The AAPM, IOMP, International Atomic Energy Agency (IAEA), and other organizations have made significant investments in education and training programmes directed towards medical physicists in LMICs [21, 22]. Several professional organizations within the radiotherapy and radiology space have, in recent times, made efforts to promote equity and inclusion within the field by the establishment of international councils. These councils, with the primary goal of increasing international collaborations to promote global standards and education in medical physics, help bridge the gap between different regions (see Chapter 2).

Organizations like the AAPM, IOMP, and the IAEA have established funded initiatives aimed at promoting gender diversity and inclusion, with the latter establishing the Marie Sklodowska-Curie Fellowship Programme [23] to bring more women into the field of nuclear and medical physics. The initiatives of equity and inclusion have also extended into equity in access to care for patients. There are current global initiatives dedicated to ensuring equitable access to medical physics services by expanding radiotherapy and diagnostic imaging services in LMICs. This has mostly been supported by international organizations and non-governmental organizations (NGOs) [24, 25]. The next few paragraphs show sample case studies of successful global collaborations that have promoted EDI in medical physics at the time of writing this book chapter. Note that Chapter 17 provides an additional list of global collaboration organizations.

16.4.1 Case Studies

16.4.1.1 Medical Physics for World Benefit (MPWB) [26]

With the growing burden of cancer worldwide and most especially in communities and regions that are underserved [27], institutions and organizations including the MPWB made it their mission over the last decade to be a part of the solution through volunteer-based activities to provide education and training for medical physics professionals. Since 2015, the organization has worked on developing a publicly accessible resource for medical physics radiation oncology training the "MPWB open syllabus project" with the intention to connect freely accessible online materials, such as presentations, documents, reports, videos, and other educational media directly with the components of the IAEA TC-37 report [28] of training requirements for medical physics residents specializing in radiation oncology. This MPWB resource shares similarities with other medical physics residency training documents, such as those found in CAMPEP [29] and other residency training syllabi [30]. The goal of this open-access resource is primarily to help medical physics residents, particularly in LMICs, gain access to curated freely accessible resources. In addition to this, the MPWB in collaboration with industry partners provides funding for physicists practising in limited resource countries to attend virtually the annual AAPM conference, providing an avenue for these individuals to participate in a conference which would otherwise have been too expensive to attend.

16.4.1.2 The Abdus Salam International Centre for Theoretical Physics (ICTP)/IAEA Sandwich Training Education Programme (STEP)

The ICTP/IAEA STEP programme has offered numerous fellowships to PhD students from LMICs with the goal of strengthening the scientific capabilities of early career scientists and researchers to better contribute to the development of their home countries. The STEP programme is structured to give each student access to the ICTP and IAEA facilities through financially supporting them for three, six-month stays each year for up to three successive years. The fellows work with advisors from their home countries and co-advisors from the host institutions. In addition to the STEP programme, ICTP regularly organizes workshops and programmes targeted mainly at scientists from developing countries, including a two-year Master of Advanced Studies in Medical Physics [31].

16.4.1.3 The Rayos Contra Cancer (RCC)

Since 2019 the RCC has completed 29 virtual training programmes [32–34] with over 2,000 participants from over 500 unique radiotherapy centres in 54 countries. These programmes are hour-long sessions that include didactic, question-and-answer dialogue with participants and practice cases. An example of EDI inclusion is the organization's evolutionary approach to accounting for a more diverse time zone and the awareness of the heterogeneity amongst participants' prior knowledge and access to different equipment and vendor types. This led to the creation of more educational content with language translation, live interpreters, and sought out moderators with diverse language skills and cultural backgrounds. Additionally, accounting for the diversity in radiotherapy equipment had led to the refinement of the educational content making it vendor-neutral. The RCC case study shows an organization's approach to bridging the equity gap in radiotherapy by maintaining a positive, productive, and inclusive environment of cultural and clinical differences to improve educational gaps.

16.5 STRATEGIES FOR PROMOTING EDI IN GLOBAL MEDICAL PHYSICS

With the remarkable work being done across various organizations, it is vital that these institutions continue to champion EDI in medical physics – particularly in the current climate where programmes dedicated to EDI efforts are frequently under attack [35]. We must advocate for more inclusive educational programmes, equitable distribution of funding, and prioritize international collaborations, especially from regions underrepresented in scientific research. Capacity building remains a powerful avenue to drive progress. One such initiative is the Cancer Research Education Excellence in Radiotherapy (CaREER) programme, part of the Comprehensive Cancer Centre in the Cloud (C4) platform [36]. This programme is designed to train a highly diverse next generation of scientists, technologists, and physicians, equipping them to pursue innovative research in radiotherapy and create cost-effective solutions to improve the quality of life for cancer patients. Participants bring a wide range of research interests, including radio-immunotherapy, FLASH radiotherapy (RT), artificial intelligence (AI), epigenetics, radiomics, nanoparticles and smart biomaterials, MRI-guided RT, and novel approaches to addressing global healthcare disparities. For participants conducting international research, co-mentors from international sites will support and enhance their experiences, leading to joint research dissemination. As part of capacity building, it is essential to leverage technology and innovation to promote EDI. Emerging technologies like telemedicine, online education platforms, and AI offer transformative possibilities for global medical physics. One successful example is the use of virtual reality to bridge the gap in brachytherapy training in underserved regions globally [37, 38].

16.6 SUMMARY AND RECOMMENDATIONS

16.6.1 Summary

It is the shared responsibility of the medical physics community to promote EDI by supporting programmes and initiatives that have the potential to enhance medical physics practice globally and improve patient care. This chapter addresses issues related to EDI in global medical physics milieu by placing it in a historical context and looking at the challenges and possible solutions. Specific case histories are highlighted by way of example as to how we can move forward. To create an equitable and inclusive global research and professional community in medical physics, where all individuals have equal access to opportunities for education, research, and professional development, we need to foster diversity in ideas and background, and in this context regardless of geographic and socioeconomic boundaries, to drive innovation in medical physics. Through cross-continent collaboration, we can continue to aim to empower a diverse medical physics workforce ensuring that innovative outcomes are beneficial to all patients including those in underrepresented and underserved regions, addressing global health challenges, and reducing disparities in health outcomes. The following recommendations provide examples of key areas that need continued investment.

16.6.2 Recommendations

1. **Medical Physics Education:** Provide support for programmes that increase access to medical physics education and training in LMICs to ensure that medical physicists from all regions of the world can contribute as well as benefit from the field.

2. **EDI Education:** Provide education in all settings on EDI solutions through conference symposia, seminars, webinars, residency, and mentorship programmes. See for example the journal club initiative [39].

3. **Research:** Promote diversity in clinical and translational research in addition to technology development and adaptation amongst diverse

clinical settings. This will ensure that advances in medical physics are relevant and beneficial for everyone.

4. **Workforce Development**: Build a workforce with a range of backgrounds and perspectives. This will improve innovation, critical thinking, and produce professionals who are culturally competent to provide patient care.

5. **Cross-Cultural Collaboration:** Promote collaborations between high-income countries and LMICs in research and clinical practices, to foster mutual growth and the development of culturally appropriate solutions.

REFERENCES

1. Pollard-Larkin JM, Roth TM, Seuntjens J, *et al.* Equity, Diversity, and Inclusion Are Essential in Medical Physics. *Int J Radiat Oncol Biol Phys.* 2023;116(2):290–294.
2. Hendrickson KRG, Avery SM, Castillo R, *et al.* 2021 AAPM Equity, Diversity, and Inclusion Climate Survey Executive Summary. *Int J Radiat Oncol Biol Phys.* 2023;116(2):295–304.
3. Elzawawy AM. Could African and Low- and Middle-Income Countries Contribute Scientifically to Global Cancer Care? *J Global Oncol.* 2015;1(2):49–53.
4. de Souza JA, Hunt BR, Asirwa FC, Adebamowo CA, Lopes GdL. Global Health Equity: Cancer Care Outcome Disparities in High-, Middle-, and Low-Income Countries. *J Clin Oncol.* 2016;34 1:6–13.
5. Xie Y, Zhang C, Lai Q. China's Rise as a Major Contributor to Science and Technology. *Proc Natl Acad Sci USA.* 2014;111(26):9437–9442.
6. Kumar D. Developing a History of Science and Technology in South Asia. *Econ Polit Weekly.* 2003;38(23):2248–2251.
7. Christ SM, Willmann J. Measuring Global Inequity in Radiation Therapy: Resource Deficits in Low- and Middle-Income Countries Without Radiation Therapy Facilities. *Adv Radiat Oncol.* 2023;8(4):101175.
8. Lawson MB, Scheel JR, Onega T, Carlos RC, Lee CI. Tackling Health Disparities in Radiology: A Practical Conceptual Framework. *J Am Coll Radiol.* 2022;19(2 Pt B):344–347.
9. Baird CL. Male-Dominated Stem Disciplines: How Do We Make Them More Attractive to Women? IEEE *Instrum Measure Mag.* 2018;21(3):4–14.
10. Francis B, Archer L, Moote J, DeWitt J, MacLeod E, Yeomans L. The Construction of Physics as a Quintessentially Masculine Subject: Young People's Perceptions of Gender Issues in Access to Physics. *Sex Roles.* 2017;76(3):156–174.
11. Covington EL, Moran JM, Paradis KC. The State of Gender Diversity in Medical Physics. *Med Phys.* 2020;47(4):2038–2043.

12. Pollard-Larkin JM, Paradis KC, Moran JM, Martel MK, Rong Y. Voices for Gender Equity in Medical Physics. *J Appl Clin Med Phys*. 2018;19(6):6–10.

13. van Zyl M, Haynes EMK, Batchelar D, Jakobi JM. Examining Gender Diversity Growth as a Model For Inclusion of All Underrepresented Persons in Medical Physics. *Med Phys*. 2020;47(12):5976–5985.

14. Paradis KC, Moran JM, Hendrickson KRG. Women in Medical Physics. *Med Phys*. 2023;50(S1):80–84.

15. McCoy D, Kapilashrami A, Kumar R, Rhule E, Khosla R. Developing an Agenda for the Decolonization of Global Health. *Bull World Health Organ*. 2024;102(2):130–136.

16. Kwete X, Tang K, Chen L, *et al*. Decolonizing Global Health: What Should Be the Target of This Movement and Where Does It Lead Us? *Global Health Res Policy*. 2022;7(1):3.

17. DeCamp M, Matandika L, Chinula L, *et al*. Decolonizing Global Health Research: Perspectives from US and International Global Health Trainees. *Ann Glob Health*. 2023;89(1):9.

18. Omofoye TS. Radiology Education as a Global Health Service Vehicle. *Radiol Imaging Cancer*. 2022;4(6):e220156.

19. Frija G, Blažić I, Frush DP, *et al*. How to Improve Access to Medical Imaging in Low- and Middle-Income Countries? *EClinicalMedicine*. 2021;38:101034.

20. Hricak H, Abdel-Wahab M, Atun R, *et al*. Medical Imaging and Nuclear Medicine: A Lancet Oncology Commission. *Lancet Oncol*. 2021;22(4):e136–e172.

21. International Atomic Energy Agency (IAEA). *Guidelines for the Certification of Clinically Qualified Medical Physicists*. IAEA, Vienna; 2021.

22. Parker SA, Weygand J, Bernat BG, *et al*. Assessing Radiology and Radiation Therapy Needs for Cancer Care in Low-and-Middle-Income Countries: Insight from a Global Survey of Departmental and Institutional Leaders. *Adv Radiat Oncol*. 2024;9(11):101615.

23. International Atomic Energy Agency (IAEA). The IAEA Marie Skłodowska-Curie Fellowship Programme: Scholarships with Internships for More Women in Nuclear. https://www.iaea.org/services/key-programmes/together-for-more-women-in-nuclear/iaea-marie-sklodowska-curie-fellowship-programme. [Accessed 2025-02-11]

24. Li B, Castaneda SA, Sherry AD, *et al*. The Implementation of Rayos Contra Cancer: Beginning a Global Health Social Enterprise. *Int J Radiat Oncol Biol Phys*. 2019;105(1):E443–E444.

25. Van Dyk, J PY, White G, Wilkins D, Basran P, Jeraj R. Medical Physics for World Benefit (MPWB): A Not-for-Profit, Volunteer Organization in Support of Medical Physics in Lower Income Environments. *Med Phys Int*. 2018;6:152–155.

26. Medical Physics for World Benefit (MPWB). www.mpwb.org. [Accessed 2025-02-11]

27. Bray F, Jemal A, Grey N, Ferlay J, Forman D. Global Cancer Transitions According to the Human Development Index (2008–2030): A Population-Based Study. *Lancet Oncol*. 2012;13(8):790–801.

28. International Atomic Energy Agency (IAEA). *Clinical Training of Medical Physicists Specializing in Radiation Oncology.* IAEA, Vienna; 2010.

29. Commission on Accreditation of Medical Physics Education Programs IC. Standards for Accreditation of Residency Educational Programs in Medical Physics, Revised July 2024. https://campep.org/. [Accessed 2025-02-11]

30. Garibaldi C, Essers M, Heijmen B, *et al.* The 3rd ESTRO-EFOMP Core Curriculum for Medical Physics Experts in Radiotherapy. *Radioth Oncol.* 2022;170:89–94.

31. International Center for Theoretical Physics (ICTP). Master of Advanced Studies in Medical Physics. https://www.ictp.it/opportunity/master-advanced-studies-medical-physics. [Accessed 2025-02-11]

32. Yorke AA, Carlson C, Koufigar S, Zhu H, Li B. Reimagining Education in Global Radiotherapy: The Experiences and Contribution of Rayos Contra Cancer. *JCO Glob Oncol.* 2023;9:e2200320.

33. Hatcher JB, Oladeru O, Chang B, *et al.* Impact of High-Dose-Rate Brachytherapy Training via Telehealth in Low- and Middle-Income Countries. *JCO Glob Oncol.* 2020;6:1803–1812.

34. Balbach ML, Neely G, Yorke A, *et al.* Developing an Educational "Hub": Impact of a Distance-Learning Curriculum in a Multinational Cohort. *BMC Med Educ.* 2024;24(1):406.

35. Blackstock OJ, Isom JE, Legha RK. Health Care is the New Battlefront for Anti-DEI Attacks. *PLOS Glob Public Health.* 2024;4(4):e0003131.

36. Cancer Research Education Excellence in Radiotherapy (CaREER), Available at: https://c4career.org/career/. [Accessed 2025-02-14].

37. Prabhu AV, Peterman M, Kesaria A, Samanta S, Crownover R, Lewis GD. Virtual Reality Technology: A Potential Tool to Enhance Brachytherapy Training and Delivery. *Brachytherapy.* 2023;22(6):709–715.

38. Taunk NK, Shah NK, Hubley E, Anamalayil S, Trotter JW, Li T. Virtual Reality-Based Simulation Improves Gynecologic Brachytherapy Proficiency, Engagement, and Trainee Self-Confidence. *Brachytherapy.* 2021;20(4):695–700.

39. Fagerstrom JM, Windsor C, Zaks D. Equity, Diversity, and Inclusion Topics at a Medical Physics Residency Journal Club. *J Appl Clin Med Phys.* 2023;24(9):e14126.

CHAPTER 17

Global Collaboration Organizations

Arun Chougule and Mary Joan

17.1 CHAPTER OBJECTIVES

- To provide a broad description of the types of organizations involved in global collaborations

- To consider the pros and cons of organizational structures and activities in global collaborations

- To provide examples of organizational global collaboration activities

- To provide recommendations regarding engagement with organizations involved with global collaboration activities

17.2 INTRODUCTION

Medical physics is a multidisciplinary field that requires rigorous and comprehensive education to meet the demands of modern healthcare. The continuous advancement in medical technologies and practices necessitates that medical physics education remains current and of high quality. Achieving this requires the close collaboration of professional organizations, academic institutions, healthcare facilities, and regulatory bodies. This chapter explores the critical role of such collaborations in raising the standards of medical physics education, highlighting key initiatives, benefits, and future directions. Note that "research is a key pillar for the

DOI: 10.1201/9781003527749-17

long-term improvement of cancer control, along with clinical and education or training activities" [1]; hence, research collaborations are also addressed.

In the rapidly evolving field of medical physics, the role of global collaboration organizations has become increasingly vital by facilitating the sharing of knowledge, resources, and expertise across borders, fostering innovation and advancements in medical physics that benefit patient care worldwide. By promoting international cooperation, they address the diverse and complex challenges faced by medical physicists, ensuring that cutting-edge techniques and technologies are accessible to all regions. By way of example, Van Dyk and Meghzifene listed 34 organizations in support of enriching radiation therapy capabilities in low-resource settings [2].

This chapter delves into the various global organizations associated with medical physics, exploring their missions, structures, and the pivotal roles they play in enhancing the field as well as bridging the gap between developed and developing regions. Figure 17.1 shows a word cloud summarizing the various organizations that are considered in this chapter.

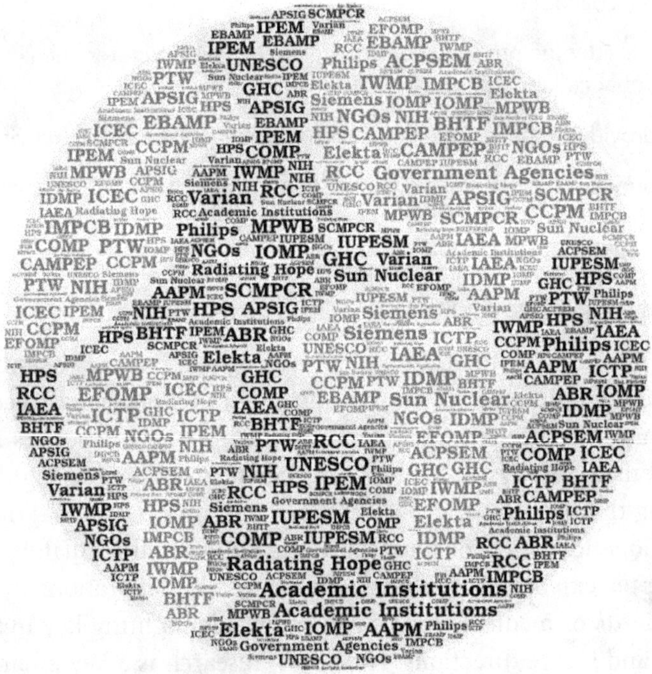

FIGURE 17.1 Various global collaboration organizations associated with medical physics as described in this chapter.

17.3 TYPES OF ORGANIZATIONS INVOLVED IN GLOBAL COLLABORATIONS

Global collaborating organizations can be broadly categorized into professional societies, academic institutions, governmental and intergovernmental agencies, non-governmental organizations (NGOs), and industry partners.

Professional societies, such as the International Organization for Medical Physics (IOMP), and regional organizations [3] along with the American Association of Physicists in Medicine (AAPM) [4], the Institute of Physics and Engineering in Medicine (IPEM) [5], Health Physics Society (HPS) [6] are at the forefront of promoting excellence in medical physics. In addition, clinical societies, such as the American Society for Radiation Oncology (ASTRO) [7] and the Radiological Society of North America (RSNA) [8], closely aligned with medical physics, provide similar international support. These societies set standards and guidelines, ensuring uniformity and quality in medical physics practices globally. Furthermore, they facilitate international educational and training activities, conferences, workshops, and webinars, providing platforms for knowledge exchange and professional networking.

Institutions like the Abdul Salam International Centre for Theoretical Physics (ICTP) [9] and the ASEAN College of Medical Physics [10] collaborate with counterparts worldwide to share advancements in medical physics, develop new technologies, and educate the next generation of medical physicists. The International Atomic Energy Agency (IAEA) [11] has been instrumental in supporting medical physics education in developing countries through its Human Health Division [12]. By providing educational resources, training programmes, and fellowships, the IAEA helps to raise the standards of medical physics education globally.

NGOs like the International Union for Physical and Engineering Sciences in Medicine (IUPESM) [13], Medical Physics for World Benefit (MPWB) [14], Radiating Hope [15], South Asian Centre for Medical Physics and Cancer Research (SCMPCR) [16], and the Better Health Technology Foundation (BHTF) [17] of Australia are promoting research and development in medical physics and promoting safe and appropriate use of medical technology. The Asia-Pacific Special Interest Group (APSIG) [18] within the field of medical physics and related healthcare professions typically focuses on promoting collaboration, education, and the advancement of medical physics in the Asia-Pacific region. Many other voluntary organizations often focus on humanitarian efforts, such as improving cancer treatment infrastructure in low- and middle-income countries (LMICs), providing training to local medical professionals, and advocating for global health equity. From a diagnostic imaging perspective, RAD-AID International [19] brings radiology to low-resource areas by delivering education, equipment, infrastructure, and support.

Medical device manufacturers and technology companies, including giants like Elekta Medical Systems [20], IBA [21], Philips Healthcare [22], PTW [23], Sun Nuclear [24], and Siemens *Healthineers*/Varian Medical Systems [25], are integral to global collaborations in medical physics by developing innovative medical technologies, offering technical training, and participating in joint research ventures, supporting education and training, ensuring that the latest advancements in medical physics are effectively translated into clinical practice worldwide.

17.3.1 Accreditation of Medical Physics Education

Accreditation is often a prerequisite for professional certification bodies, such as the American Board of Radiology (ABR) [26] or the Canadian College of Physicists in Medicine (CCPM) [27]. The IOMP has established an accreditation board which accredits master's in medical physics education programmes, structured residency programmes, and continuous professional development programmes (CPD) conducted in any part of the world. Similarly, many countries have established their own accreditation boards, e.g., the Commission on Accreditation of Medical Physics Educational Programmes (CAMPEP) [28], the Australasian College of Physical Scientists and Engineers in Medicine (ACPSEM) [29], the Institute of Physics and Engineering in Medicine (IPEM) are to mention a few. The Canadian Organization of Medical Physicists (COMP) [30] promotes the development of standards, policies, guidelines, and research related to medical physics. EFOMP [31] works to harmonize the standards of education and training in medical physics across Europe and established the European Board of Accreditation for Medical Physics (EBAMP) [32]. IOMP has established the International Medical Physics Certification Board (IMPCB) [33] which accredits national certification boards and provides individual certification of medical physicists where such boards do not exist.

17.3.2 Pros and Cons of Organizational Structures and Activities in Global Collaborations

17.3.2.1 Pros

Global collaborations in medical physics involve various organizational structures and activities, each with its own advantages and disadvantages. Understanding these can help optimize collaborations and address challenges effectively.

Professional societies establish and disseminate standards and guidelines, ensuring consistent practices and high-quality care globally. They provide platforms for professionals to network, share knowledge, and stay updated on the latest developments through conferences and workshops. Societies offer certifications, training programmes, and continuous education opportunities, enhancing the skills and competencies of medical physicists. Academic institutions provide high-quality education and training programmes to drive innovation through research, leading to advancements in medical physics technologies and methodologies. They often engage in international research collaborations, fostering the exchange of ideas and expertise. Governmental and intergovernmental agencies have significant financial resources to support large-scale projects and initiatives. They provide essential regulatory frameworks and policies that ensure the safe and effective use of medical physics technologies. Nongovernmental agencies support capacity-building initiatives in developing countries, enhancing local capabilities in medical physics. NGOs often target their efforts towards underserved regions, addressing disparities in medical physics services to improve cancer treatment in LMICs. Industry partners drive technological advancements, providing state-of-the-art equipment and solutions by offering technical training and support to medical physicists. They engage in research and development collaborations, pushing the boundaries of medical physics applications.

17.3.2.2 Cons

Some societies may face a shortage of experienced leaders and financial constraints, limiting their ability to support large-scale initiatives. While professional organizations aim for global reach, their benefits may be more accessible to members in developed regions. Research projects often depend on uncertain external funding, and academic institutions may encounter bureaucratic delays. Governmental processes and changing policies can also slow project implementation.

NGOs rely on unpredictable donations, while industry partners may prioritize profitable markets over broader goals. Despite these challenges, each organization involved in global medical physics collaborations brings valuable strengths. By leveraging these strengths and mitigating the challenges, they can enhance their collective impact, advancing medical physics and improving global healthcare outcomes.

17.4 EXAMPLES OF ORGANIZATIONAL GLOBAL COLLABORATION ACTIVITIES

The IOMP organizes the triennial World Congress on Medical Physics and Biomedical Engineering bringing together thousands of professionals from around the world to share research, discuss advancements, and foster international collaborations.

The IOMP's International Day of Medical Physics and the International Medical Physics Week, celebrated annually, raise awareness about the role of medical physicists and promote the exchange of knowledge through workshops, webinars, and public lectures.

The Harvard Medical School – Global Health Catalyst Summit [34] focuses on leveraging telemedicine to improve cancer care in low-resource settings, bringing together academic researchers, healthcare providers, and industry partners to discuss innovative solutions.

The University of Sydney – Medical Physics and Radiation Oncology Research Group [35] and similar research groups at various universities across the world collaborate with international institutions to conduct research on advanced radiation therapy techniques, contributing to global (https://rad-aid.org/) advancements in cancer treatment.

The IAEA's Human Health Campus [36] offers online training, guidelines, and courses for medical physicists, improving radiation safety and medical imaging quality. It supports developing countries by enhancing medical physics infrastructure, establishing radiotherapy centres, and training local professionals through the Technical Cooperation Programme. The IAEA also lists global collaboration organizations [37], leading to joint research, exchange programmes, and co-authored publications, enriching global knowledge.

The ICTP organizes specialized workshops and schools in medical physics, offering participants from developing countries training in advanced radiation therapy, medical imaging, and other essential healthcare areas. It provides fellowships and associateships to facilitate collaborative research, bridging the gap between developed and developing regions. In collaboration with the University of Trieste and over 20 hospitals, the ICTP runs a Master's of Advanced Studies in Medical Physics (MMP) programme for candidates from underserved regions like Africa, Latin America, and Eastern Europe.

The US National Institutes of Health (NIH) [38] funds and coordinates international research collaborations to address global health challenges, including cancer and other diseases where medical physics plays a crucial role.

Radiating Hope collects and donates radiotherapy equipment to hospitals in low-income countries, improving their capacity to treat cancer patients, and organizes workshops to train local medical professionals in the use of donated equipment and advanced treatment techniques.

The International Cancer Expert Corps (ICEC) [39] connects experienced medical physicists and oncologists with professionals in developing countries, providing mentorship and support to improve local cancer care services.

Rayos Contra Cancer (RCC) [40] gives very practical courses on specific radiation therapy techniques, especially in LMICs, largely via digital technologies [41].

Medical Physics for World Benefit (MPWB) [14] supports activities that yield effective and safe use of physics and technologies in medicine through advising, training, demonstrating, and/or participating in medical physics-related activities, especially in LMICs by leveraging the expertise and technology in medical physics to address global health challenges and improve healthcare outcomes worldwide.

The Global Training Academy of Siemens Healthineers partners with academic and clinical institutions worldwide to develop and test new medical physics technologies and applications.

Access to Care programmes of Varian Medical Systems aims to expand access to radiotherapy in underserved regions by providing affordable equipment and training local medical professionals and collaborates with hospitals to advance the availability of cutting-edge cancer treatment modalities.

These are only some examples and illustrate the diverse and impactful activities that organizations engage in to foster global collaboration in medical physics. By combining resources, expertise, and innovative approaches, these collaborations contribute significantly to advancing the field and improving healthcare outcomes worldwide.

17.5 SUMMARY AND RECOMMENDATIONS

17.5.1 Summary

This chapter explores the significant role of global collaboration organizations in the field of medical physics. Such organizations can be broadly categorized as professional societies, academic institutions, governmental and intergovernmental agencies, non-governmental organizations (NGOs), and industry partners. Such organizations foster international cooperation, promote educational and professional standards, facilitate research and development, and are a vital resource for advancing education and research, especially in LMIC contexts.

17.5.2 Recommendations Related to Medical Physics Organizations

1. Medical physics organizations involved in education and training are encouraged to increase participation from developing countries through scholarships and grants to expand funding opportunities for students and professionals from LMICs.

2. Professional societies should encourage virtual participation options for conferences and workshops through remote access.

3. Professional medical physics organizations should foster interdisciplinary collaboration by joint initiatives between medical physicists and professionals from related fields such as radiology, oncology, and biomedical engineering.

4. International collaborative organizations and regional societies should create forums for interdisciplinary dialogue and project development.

5. Professional organizations should take initiatives to standardize education and certification by developing a standardized curriculum for medical physics education recognized internationally and promoting a unified certification process to ensure consistent professional standards.

6. Academic institutions and governmental and non-governmental organizations should enhance research collaboration by establishing global research networks to tackle common health issues and technological challenges and facilitate the sharing of research data and findings across borders.

7. All stakeholders of medical physics should promote sustainable practices and green initiatives by encouraging the adoption of sustainable practices in medical physics research and clinical applications and trying to bring down the carbon footprint of each and every associated activity. The first step towards this could be resource optimization by developing strategies for the efficient use of resources, especially in low-resource settings.

8. Medical physicists and their professional organizations should take part in strengthening communication and outreach by increasing public awareness of the role and impact of medical physics in healthcare and by improving communication between global organizations to align goals and strategies, and to avoid duplication of effort.

9. International collaborative organizations, industry partners, and national and regional medical physics professional bodies should support continuous professional development through ongoing training and mentorship programmes.

10. Global medical physics organizations should enhance their impact by ensuring equitable access to education and resources and fostering a unified and effective global medical physics community.

17.5.3 Recommendations for Medical Physicists

Engaging with organizations involved in global collaboration activities in medical physics can be highly beneficial for professional development, networking, and contributing to the advancement of the field. For effectively engaging with these organizations, the first step is to identify the key organizations and become familiar with leading organizations in medical physics that have a global focus. Joining these organizations may provide access to member benefits, such as networking opportunities with professionals worldwide; access to journals, publications, and research; discounts on conferences and workshops, continuing education and certification programmes.

Volunteering for committees, working groups, or task forces within these organizations allows an influence in the direction of global initiatives, collaboration on international projects, and gain leadership experience and recognition. Here are some suggestions for active global collaborations:

1. Engage in collaborative research projects and clinical trials facilitated by these organizations to have access to diverse datasets and resources, opportunities for co-authoring publications with international researchers, and for enhancing the impact and reach of research.

2. Focus on the development and dissemination of affordable and robust medical technologies suitable for low-resource settings such as low-cost imaging equipment, portable radiation therapy devices, and telemedicine solutions for remote diagnostics and consultations.

3. Take advantage of training programmes, webinars, online courses, and open-access educational resources and materials offered by these organizations. This can help to stay updated with the latest practices and technologies, fulfil continuing education requirements, and to enhance skills in specialized areas of medical physics.

4. Use platforms provided by these organizations to network and connect with professionals. Strategies include joining online forums and discussion groups, participating in social media groups and activities, and engaging in mentorship programmes as a mentor or mentee.

5. Share or contribute expertise by writing articles or opinion pieces for organizational newsletters and journals, speaking at conferences or webinars, and serving as a peer reviewer for publications.

6. Participate in or organize volunteer missions to provide medical physics expertise in disaster-stricken or underserved areas by setting up temporary diagnostic and treatment facilities, training local healthcare workers, and providing technical support and maintenance for medical equipment.

7. Advocate for policies that promote global health equity and the integration of medical physics into health systems worldwide by collaborating with global health policy-makers, participating in advocacy campaigns, and writing policy briefs and position statements.

8. Encourage and implement sustainable practices in medical physics to reduce environmental impact by reducing the use of hazardous materials, promoting energy-efficient technologies, and supporting recycling and proper disposal of medical equipment.

9. Keep yourself updated with the latest news, developments, and opportunities from these organizations by subscribing to newsletters, following on social media, and regularly visiting websites.

By actively engaging with organizations involved in global collaboration in medical physics, one can significantly contribute to the field's growth while also enhancing one's own professional development. Individuals who choose to follow some of these recommendations can significantly contribute to improving global health outcomes and ensuring that advanced medical technologies and expertise are accessible to all.

REFERENCES

1. Abdel-Wahab, M., et al., Global Radiotherapy: Current Status and Future Directions-White Paper. JCO Glob Oncol, 2021. 7: p. 827–842.
2. Van Dyk, J. and A. Meghzifene, Radiation Oncology Quality and Safety Considerations in Low-Resource Settings: A Medical Physics Perspective. Semin Radiat Oncol, 2017. 27(2): p. 124–135.
3. International Organization for Medical Physics (IOMP). IOMP Regional Organizations. [Accessed 2024-08-21]; Available from: https://www.iomp.org/regional-organizations/.

4. American Association of Physicists in Medicine (AAPM). [Accessed 2024-08-21]; Available from: https://w4.aapm.org/org/.

5. Institute of Physics and Engineering in Medicine (IPEM). [Accessed 2024-08-21]; Available from: https://www.ipem.ac.uk/.

6. Health Physics Society (HPS). [Accessed 2024-08-21]; Available from: https://hps.org/.

7. American Society of Radiation Oncology (ASTRO). [Accessed 2025-02-17]; Available from: https://www.astro.org/.

8. Radiological Society of North America (RSNA). [Accessed 2025-02-17]; Available from: https://www.rsna.org/.

9. International Centre for Theoretical Physics (ICTP). [Accessed 2024-08-21]; Available from: https://www.ictp.it/.

10. ASEAN College of Medical Physics. [Accesssed 2024-08-21]; Available from: https://seafomp.org/acomp/.

11. International Atomic Energy Agency (IAEA). [Accessed 2024-08-21]; Available from: https://www.iaea.org/.

12. International Atomic Energy Agency (IAEA). Division of Human Health. [Accessed 2024-08-21]; Available from: https://www.iaea.org/about/organizational-structure/department-of-nuclear-sciences-and-applications/division-of-human-health.

13. International Union for Physical and Engineering Sciences in Medicine (IUPESM). [Accessed 2024-08-21]; Available from: https://iupesm.org/.

14. Medical Physics for World Benefit. [Accessed 2024-08-21]; Available from: www.mpwb.org.

15. Radiating Hope. [Accessed 2024-08-21]; Available from: https://www.radiatinghope.org/.

16. South Asian Centre for Medical Physics and Cancer Research (SCMPCR). [Accessed 2024-08-21]; Available from: https://scmpcr.org/.

17. Better Health Technology Foundation (BHTF). [Accessed 2024-08-21]; Available from: https://www.betterhealthcaretechnology.org/.

18. Asia-Pacific Special Interest Group (APSIG). [Accessed 2024-08-21]; Available from: https://www.betterhealthcaretechnology.org/apsig/.

19. RAD-AID International. [Accessed 2025-02-17]; Available from: https://rad-aid.org/.

20. Elekta. [Accessed 2024-08-21]; Available from: https://www.elekta.com/.

21. IBA. [Accessed 2024-08-21]; Available from: https://www.iba-worldwide.com/.

22. Philips Healthcare. [Accessed 2024-08-21]; Available from: https://www.usa.philips.com/healthcare/.

23. PTW. [Accessed 2024-08-21]; Available from: https://www.ptwdosimetry.com/en/.

24. Sun Nuclear. [Accessed 2024-08-21]; Available from: https://www.ptwdosimetry.com/en/.

25. Siemens Healthineers/Varian Medical Systems. [Accessed 2024-08-21]; Available from: https://www.varian.com/.

26. American Board of Radiology (ABR). [Accessed 2024-08-21]; Available from: https://www.theabr.org/.
27. Canadian College of Physicists in Medicine (CCPM). [Accessed 2024-08-21]; Available from: https://ccpm.ca/.
28. Commission on Accreditation of Medical Physics Education Programs (CAMPEP). [Accessed 2024-08-21]; Available from: http://campep.org/.
29. Australasian College of Physical Scientists and Engineers in Medicine (ACPSEM). [Accessed 2024-08-21]; Available from: https://www.acpsem.org.au/Home.
30. Canadian Organization of Medical Physicists (COMP). [Accessed 2024-08-21]; Available from: https://comp-ocpm.ca/.
31. European Federation of Organisations for Medical Physics (EFOMP). [Accessed 2024-08-21]; Available from: https://www.efomp.org/.
32. European Board of Accreditation for Medical Physics (EBAMP). [Accessed 2024-08-21]; Available from: https://www.ebamp.eu/.
33. International Medical Physics Certification Board (IMPCB). [Accessed 2024-08-21]; Available from: http://www.impcbdb.org/.
34. Global Health Catalyst Summit. [Accesssed 2024-08-21]; Available from: https://www.globalhealthcatalystsummit.org/.
35. University of Sydney - Medical Physics and Radiation Oncology Research Group. [Accessed 2024-08-21]; Available from: https://www.sydney.edu.au/science/our-research/research-centres/institute-of-medical-physics.html.
36. International Atomic Energy Agency (IAEA). Human Health Campus. [Accessed 2024-08-21]; Available from: https://www.iaea.org/resources/databases/human-health-campus.
37. International Atomic Energy Agency (IAEA). Organizations for Global Collaborations in Medical Physics. [Accessed 204-08-21]; Available from: https://www.iaea.org/resources/hhc/medical-physics/ongoing-collaborations.
38. US National Institutes of Health (NIH). [Accessed 2024-08-21]; Available from: https://www.nih.gov/.
39. International Cancer Expert Corps (ICEC). [Accessed 2024-08-21]; Available from: https://www.iceccancer.org/.
40. Rayos Contra Cancer (RCC). [Accessed 2024-08-21]; Available from: https://www.rayoscontracancer.org/.
41. Rayos Contra Cancer (RCC). Training Programs. [Accessed 2024-08-21]; Available from: https://www.rayoscontracancer.org/training-programs.

CHAPTER 18

International Collaborations: Summary and Recommendations

Jacob Van Dyk

18.1 CHAPTER OBJECTIVES

- To summarize highlights of global collaborations as discussed in earlier chapters

- To summarize recommendations discussed in earlier chapters

18.2 SUMMARY: INTERNATIONAL GLOBAL COLLABORATIONS

Participation in global medical physics activities has the potential for generating a range of emotions, often shaped by project outcomes. For successful projects where patient care or education advancement is improved, these emotions can provide a deep sense of accomplishment providing incentives for further engagement. However, where projects falter or do not provide the hoped for outcomes, they provide a sense of frustration and disappointment that discourages the good work of global medical physics activities. It is the hope that the multiple chapters of this book have provided an educational aid that will help medical physicists interested in

DOI: 10.1201/9781003527749-18

global health activities to sway the pendulum on the side of success and to minimize the possibilities of failure.

Personal	• Interest in global health: ▸ Why? How? When? Where? • Aim: ▸ To reduce disparities, To develop technologies, To advance research
Collaboration	• With whom? • Collaboration in: ▸ Clinical service, Teaching/Training, Research • Readiness • Preparation • Education/training for global involvement • Engage/buy-in at highest level partners • Principles of: ▸ Humility, Mutual respect, Solidarity, Social justice • Awareness of collaborative organizations
Project Preparation	• Needs assessment: ▸ Local needs ■ Major driver, Set by locals, Abide by local standards/regulations • Goals • Scope • Awareness: ▸ Communication channels ■ How, Who, Hierarchy, Language, Cultural sensitivity, Ethical behaviour, Confidentiality, Transparency, Humility, Respect, Honesty, Accountability • Training for global medical physics activities: ▸ Volunteers/contributors, Hosts • Leverage professional and other organizations • Develop measures of outcome/impact
Project Planning	• Organizational capacity: ▸ Consensus led, Common passions, Flat hierarchy, Light managerial/organizational structure • Strong partnerships • Project champion • Political support • Sustainability (>10 years): ▸ Human resources, Finances, Technical support • Open communication • Outcome metrics
Project Execution	• Training needs: ▸ Local, Virtual mentoring/training • Note potential barriers due to power imbalances: ▸ Language, Cultural, Ethical • Foster spirit of inclusivity/diversity • Data sharing: ▸ Clear definition, Data pre-processing needs, Apply FAIR principles (Ch. 13), Share credit
Post-Project Execution	• Review project success • Advocacy: ▸ Promote international collaborations, Enhance diplomacy, Leverage technology/media promotion, Serve on advisory boards/commissions, Advocate for global health equity, Encourage sustainable practice • Share expertise: ▸ Publications, Opinion pieces, Newsletters, Conferences, Webinars, Journal reviewer • Engagement: ▸ Collaborative research/clinical trials/diverse datasets/resources, Encourage co-authoring of publications, Take advantage of training programs/webinars/on-line courses/open access resources, Use platforms to network/connect via social media/mentorship

FIGURE 18.1 Summary of key topics regarding global medical physics, which were discussed by contributing authors in earlier chapters of the book.

It is not easy to summarize the range of information provided in earlier chapters. However, a grand summary highlighting many of the topics discussed by the contributing authors is shown in Figure 18.1. It's done in point format and divided into six major categories. It begins with the personal introspection as to why and how one would want to get involved in global collaborations, moves on to collaboration considerations, then addresses factors to consider in the actual projects, planning the projects, executing the projects, and finally to post-project considerations. All the topics listed are addressed in detail throughout the various chapters of this book.

In summary, engagement in global medical physics activities can provide a range of rewards from personal fulfilment and satisfaction to improvements in patient care and to successful collaborations with colleagues from other parts of the world. With the aid of well-structured and well-coordinated global medical physics activities, medical physicists can instil confidence and hope for further successful outcomes in future collaborations.

Index

H

I

For Product Safety Concerns and Information please contact our EU
representative GPSR@taylorandfrancis.com
Taylor & Francis Verlag GmbH, Kaufingerstraße 24, 80331 München, Germany

9 781032 864891